Whose Health Is It, Anyway?

T0177672

Whose Health Is It, Anyway?

PROFESSOR DAME SALLY C. DAVIES,
GCB, DBE, FRS, FMED SCI
Master, Trinity College Cambridge, UK

DR JONATHAN PEARSON-STUTTARD, FRSPH
Wellcome Trust Clinical Research Fellow, Imperial College London, UK

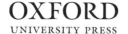
OXFORD
UNIVERSITY PRESS

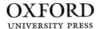

Great Clarendon Street, Oxford, OX2 6DP,
United Kingdom

Oxford University Press is a department of the University of Oxford.
It furthers the University's objective of excellence in research, scholarship,
and education by publishing worldwide. Oxford is a registered trade mark of
Oxford University Press in the UK and in certain other countries

First Edition published in 2021

Impression: 1

Published in the United States of America by Oxford University Press
198 Madison Avenue, New York, NY 10016, United States of America

British Library Cataloguing in Publication Data

Data available

Library of Congress Control Number: 2020946253

ISBN 978–0–19–886345–8

DOI: 10.1093/oso/9780198863458.001.0001

Printed and bound by
CPI Group (UK) Ltd, Croydon, CR0 4YY

For Lisa and for Willem

Foreword

The health of nations has never been a more pressing concern for governments and societies around the world as it is today. Even before the pandemic began, our ageing and growing populations, living with more co-morbidities, presented significant challenges to health systems and economies globally. The costs associated with treating and managing the heightened burden of ill-health have consumed a greater share of government budgets, while the links between poor health and productivity have become an issue of increasing concern. The COVID-19 pandemic has brought all of these factors, and the inequalities across health drivers and outcomes, to the fore in the most abrupt way. At this moment of crisis, there is a necessity to be candid, and to look at these challenges differently to mitigate the worst effects of the pandemic, and to rebuild once the worst has passed. This book is therefore both timely and relevant to the single most important issue of today and tomorrow-our collective health.

Dame Sally has a life-long track record of innovation and leadership on major issues in healthcare. She pioneered the establishment of the National Institute for Health Research (NIHR), which transformed the NHS's approach to clinical research with over £1 billion of funding to foster closer collaboration between academia and health services. As England's first female Chief Medical Officer (CMO), Dame Sally has led the advocacy and awareness of Anti-Microbial Resistance (AMR). Resulting in this issue being placed on the UK National Risk Register, work she continues to contribute to as the United Kingdom Special Envoy on AMR.

In her 2018 CMO's annual report, Health 2040 - Better Health Within Reach, Dame Sally and Jonny examined what health could look like in 2040 through an aspirational lens grounded in evidence, and in turn, what adaptions to our healthcare systems might be needed to realise this. The recommendation for a composite 'Health Index' was the first of its kind in attempting to reposition how governments view health – namely as an asset to our nation. This book, born out of the ideas and vision in that report, goes much further in seeking to address the major issues we face together today.

Throughout all nine chapters of this book a unique analysis of the challenges facing the public's health today is presented, furnished with examples, illustrations and innovative proposals for moving forward and transforming our health. Fresh insights into why our health matters to each of us both individually and collectively as society, are put forward - although we are living longer, more of these years are spent in poor health and this will continue to impact more people in years to come. In characteristic style, they harness a vision for positive change by going much further than just diagnosing the problem; they dissect the drivers (making the point that our health is not inevitable, these are not 'determinants') of the wider health environment through novel approaches. This encompasses well described social drivers of health, to more novel commercial drivers of health, capturing both how they drive the world and the environment that we live in. They also draw on the positive commercial drivers of old as demonstrated throughout the COVID-19 pandemic. The third section of the book focuses on the healthcare system. Their vision of transforming healthcare systems from 'importers of illness to exporters of health' is supported by the compelling case of the potential reward in achieving this goal, and the imperative to do so, alongside pragmatic, yet innovative, approaches that embrace emerging technologies and data analytics.

Having made the case that health is 'our most untapped opportunity for prosperity and fairness', as individuals, employers and nations, Dame Sally and Jonny close by posing the question 'Whose health is it, anyway?' Their compelling conclusion that we all must 'value health' differently is both prescient and powerful. The framework they propose to achieve this across the health ecosystem, including the wider health environment and the healthcare system – is thought provoking and forward looking in equal measure, providing much food for thought for policy makers around the world.

Professor the Lord Darzi of Denham OM KBE PC FRS
Co-Director, Institute of Global Health Innovation,
Imperial College London

Acknowledgements

The idea to write this book originated from Dame Sally's Annual Report of the Chief Medical Officer 2018, *Health 2040–Better Health Within Reach*, for which Jonny was Editor-in-Chief. The report aimed to give an ambitious vision of what the future of health could be, grounded in evidence. The report, published in December 2018, included 15 chapters, 14 of them being authored by external contributors across academia, policy, and industry from around the world. Along with several workshops and dozens of interviews, these chapters provided the framing for our core thesis of this book—that far from being a cost, or drain on society, health is our greatest untapped opportunity for prosperity and happiness in the 21st century. We thank all of the authors of chapters and case studies as well as our colleagues in the CMO's office for their work and support in the development of that report.

Developing and writing this book has allowed us to think beyond our immediate next steps for health, and our current crises and challenges to imagine what could be possible if society valued the opportunities that health brings. As we were writing, COVID-19 spread across the world and showed us the fragility of our health and health systems and how important both are to economies and wider society. This free-thinking has been thought provoking and we have both greatly enjoyed our discussions and debate together and with others about what health means to societies and what repositioning this could mean for the future. Jonny thanks Sally for her support and guidance throughout this project and beyond.

We thank several colleagues for their invaluable and detailed comments on draft sections of this book—particularly Martin Stewart-Weeks, Jonathan Grant, John Hood, Catherine Falconer, Roy Lilley, and Connor Rochford. The text is richer and the narrative more clear thanks to your input. We thank Kate Kirk for her work in editing and bringing this book to a conclusion over the final few weeks and Tony Holt for designing the book cover. Our immense thanks to Ara Darzi for kindly contributing the Foreword to our book and his thoughtful words.

Above all, we are grateful to our families for their tireless support and encouragement throughout this project and the work around it.

Contents

About the authors

Professor **Dame Sally C. Davies,** GCB, DBE, FRS, FMed Sci is a haematologist by training, specializing in sickle cell disease. She joined NHS Research and Development in 1998, as Regional Director for North-West Thames Region. She was appointed Director General for Research and Development in the Department of Health in 2004, serving until 2016. In that role she established the National Institute for Health Research (NIHR) in 2006 and led its development as Inaugural Director until 2016. In 2010 she was asked to be interim Chief Medical Officer (CMO), and became the CMO for England and Senior Medical Adviser to the UK Government in 2011. She was awarded a DBE in 2009 and GCB in the 2020 New Year Honours. She was elected a Fellow of the Royal Society in 2014 and a Member of the National Academy of Medicine, USA, in 2015. She has won many prizes for her work and globally is best known for her championing of the need to take action to prevent and mitigate Antimicrobial Resistance (AMR) as well as her central role in delivering the sequencing of one hundred thousand full genomes of patients in the NHS.

Dr **Jonathan Pearson-Stuttard**, FRSPH, is a public health physician and epidemiologist at Imperial College London. Since completing his medical training at the University of Oxford, he has been awarded multiple competitive clinical-academic research positions from NIHR and the Wellcome Trust. His research has two main streams spanning non-communicable disease epidemiology, using big data and simulation modelling of health, economic, and inequality outcomes to inform public health policy, and investigating the increasing multimorbidity and diversification of patients with chronic diseases such as diabetes. He was Editor-in-Chief of the Annual Report of the Chief Medical Officer 2018, *Health 2040–Better Health Within Reach*, which made several key recommendations, including the development of a Composite Health Index, which is currently being developed by the Office for National Statistics. Jonathan is also vice-Chair of the Royal Society for Public Health and Head of Health Analytics at Lane, Clark & Peacock and regularly comments in the media on a range of research and policy issues.

1
Introduction

As the final chapters of this book were being drafted, the COVID-19 pandemic had already claimed the lives of hundreds of thousands of people around the world. At the time of writing, the first wave has receded in some countries and lockdowns begin to ease, livelihoods of whole nations have been left in the balance and economic and societal progress has been halted and, in some cases, reversed.

The COVID-19 pandemic has meant that health, in the negative sense, has dominated our news cycles since early in 2020. Bulletins have announced the lives lost daily to the virus, dramatic falls in equity markets, plummeting GDP forecasts, rising unemployment, and entire industries being brought to a standstill. Hospitality, entertainment, sports, the arts, construction, and manufacturing all halted at the beginning of the pandemic, and months later, some are yet to re-start.

The dependency of the global economy upon the health of its citizens has been laid bare by COVID-19. The prosperity and happiness of communities and nations has been devastated by illness, and the fragility of society has been clearly revealed. Worse still, the glaring inequalities in lived experiences have translated into shocking differences in survival rates among different communities.

It is time to re-think how we value and address our health in a complex and interdependent world.

A fragile economic and political model

To protect the lives of citizens from COVID-19 today, leaders have been forced to gamble with tomorrow.

COVID-19 has rapidly and devastatingly demonstrated just how intertwined our health is with the world—and the economies—in which we live. GDP and short-term economic prosperity, the coveted prize for governments over past decades, have been revealed as dependent on the

Whose Health Is It, Anyway? Dame Sally C. Davies and Jonathan Pearson-Stuttard, Oxford University Press (2021).
© Oxford University Press. DOI: 10.1093/oso/9780198863458.003.0001

health of nations today and tomorrow, and politicians see their best-made plans for the economy and domestic agenda in tatters.

In addition, the disruption of industries and jobs coupled with urbanization had already affected the lives of many unequally. Where local economies had been stifled or broken up, differences in abilities and opportunities for finding alternative stable employment and income resulted in left-behind communities, particularly in rural areas and locations that were formerly manufacturing hubs.

On top of this, we are using fossil fuels, plastics, and antibiotics to the long-term detriment of our environment and planet, a poor legacy for our children and grandchildren. The Baby Boomer generation has unintentionally broken the inter-generational contract and the young of today are the first generation who cannot expect to be as, or more, comfortable than their predecessors. For many, therefore, it seems difficult to be optimistic about the future.

In the maelstrom of COVID-19, ministers have found themselves in the unenviable position of having to choose one unpalatable, and previously unthinkable, option over another, each with inherent trade-offs, the consequences of which will only become clear in the future, perhaps long after the decisions have been made.

Health systems have pivoted to focus almost entirely on coping with the pandemic, leaving many people needing tests or treatments for other conditions, such as cancer and cardiovascular disease, in limbo, and non-urgent procedures being postponed—we will only know the true and full impact of this in the coming months and years. In parallel, government borrowing has soared and expensive rescue packages have been put in place to mitigate the worst effects of the pandemic.

Alongside the economic and health challenges of COVID-19, trust in our leaders has eroded to an all-time low. We have had several examples of the so-called elite behaving dreadfully in recent years, abusing their position and rightly losing public trust. This is not new, and examples where unethical behaviour by a few individuals have had a hugely damaging effect have included the 2008 global financial crisis and the 2009 Parliamentary expenses scandal in the UK. The latter highlighted outrageous abuses of an archaic system where public money was used for private gain by Members of Parliament, including to buy an ornamental duck house and to pay for repairs to a privately owned moat.

COVID-19 has thrown up yet more examples of this type of behaviour. Senior public officials, doctors, and academics have flouted the lockdown rules that they themselves developed and insisted on. This has inevitably led the public to conclude that our leaders believe the rules do not apply to them; they are seemingly entitled to live by different rules and do not have to practice what they preach.

Not surprisingly, given these flagrant abuses of power, politicians are the least trusted profession in the UK. Even before the pandemic, an Ipsos MORI poll in November 2019 found that UK politicians in general were trusted to tell the truth by a mere 14% of the population (below advertising executives as the next worst at 17%), and government ministers were trusted by 17%, down 5% since 2018 [1].

If we cannot trust our leaders to guide us in the best of times, how can we trust them to lead us in the worst of times? The erosion of societal trust can be dangerous. A lack of trust coupled with a perception of unfairness leads to discontent and anger, which in turn can translate into populism, new nationalism, and angry groupings which often cross borders. Conversely, the same 'new power' that these groups are using to foster discontent, largely social media, can also be used for better outcomes. Collective citizen influence is on the rise as a force for good, and gives us cause for hope.

The Ipsos MORI poll that showed how little we trust our politicians also revealed that nurses are the profession most trusted to tell the truth, at 95%. Yet too often their employer, the NHS (the largest employer in the UK), becomes a political football, from Brexit and £350 million on the side of a bus to the recent general election where the NHS was the most important issue to voters, even more so than Brexit. Those working in the health sector urged politicians to stop playing fast and loose with statistics about healthcare and spend. In the 2019 UK general election campaign, for example, the chief executive of the NHS Confederation, which represents hospitals across the country, pleaded on the very first day of the campaign for politicians not to 'weaponize' the NHS.

> . . . disingenuous claims about extra funding, or promises that create unrealistic expectations, may be tempting in the heat of the election battle, but they do the health service no favours.
>
> Chris Hopson, NHS Confederation CEO

The disconnect between the public's trust in the NHS and the politicians' use of it as a short-term, vote-winning tool has shown to be yet another challenge for those on the front line coping with COVID-19.

Experiences of health were already different before COVID-19 came along

Before COVID-19, the world was generally in a better state than most people assumed. Nearly 1.2 billion fewer people lived in extreme poverty in 2015 compared with 1990 [2], and life expectancy was rising all over the world—in the UK, for example, life expectancy has increased from 69 to 81 over the past 60 years. By most measures these two parameters, poverty and life expectancy, have continued to improve.

But the figures mask two key issues, namely increasing relative inequality and long-term health conditions that impact on years lived in good health. Despite decreases in absolute numbers living in poverty, inequalities are rising and the difference between the richest and the poorest is increasing in many societies. Being in work in the UK is not a guarantee of being out of poverty. In addition, although people are living for many more years, an increasing number of these years are lived in poor health with one or more long-term conditions, or multimorbidities, that profoundly impact quality of life, even if the quantity of life is there.

The inequalities across and within societies have been brought to the fore by COVID-19. Worsening inequalities reduce communities to states of deprivation, where life expectancy, far from increasing, actually starts to decrease, where rates of smoking fail to match the general downwards trend, and where children are born into a precarious educational and social environment which impacts their chances and opportunities for the entirety of their lives.

Increases in life expectancy have led to the phenomenon of ageing populations, where the ratio of the population of working age to that of those in retirement begins to reverse, and the traditional model of today's taxes paying for today's pensions and social services starts to break down.

On top of this, longer lives are not necessarily, nor indeed frequently, healthier lives. The chances of contracting or developing a condition such as diabetes, cancer, or cardiovascular disease are higher the older you are, and are coupled with risk factors such as smoking or obesity. Although we have become better able to treat these conditions to keep people alive, we may not be able to cure or mitigate the condition to allow the sufferer to live well. The consequences are debilitating and the treatments add mounting costs to an already strapped set of services. To make matters worse, one of the key risk factors for a number of conditions, obesity, is on the rise. In the UK in 2017, nearly one third of adults were obese, and another third were overweight and at risk of becoming obese. Furthermore, women in the most deprived areas had overweight and obesity rates 11% higher than those in the least deprived areas [3]. According to the Organisation for Economic Co-operation and Development (OECD), the UK was the most obese country in Western Europe in 2015 [4].

Inequalities compound the complexities of the relationship between health and economic productivity, between quality of life and length of life, and between health-harming and health-promoting environments. Looking ahead, we cannot afford to try and address each of these issues separately, health is part of a much bigger picture.

We cannot afford to keep muddling through

We now find ourselves in a situation where there are no quick fixes. We face extraordinarily interconnected health, economic, and political issues, and the sticking plaster approach of shoring up a creaking system is not sustainable. Populations are ageing, multimorbidities are rising, care costs are increasing, and there is a lack of resilience in the system.

COVID-19 is the extreme end of illness, or absence of health, affecting our lives. But illness was regularly in the media before COVID-19, too. The cost of ill health and conditions such as obesity hit our news headlines weekly, or so it seemed, with worrying forecasts warning us of how much more it will cost to maintain a health service as our population ages, or headline-grabbing pledges by political parties to invest billions into systems that are struggling to cope with rising demand.

It was easy for such stories to become normalized and lead to the belief that we will always find a way to muddle through and be OK in the end. When we look a little closer, however, we find that the extra investment that we saw in the headlines is not to transform a service and hence our health as we might have hoped, but better likened to a extra spot of paint, covering over the cracks for today, in the hope of services continuing, or at least surviving, for now.

Politicians of all parties have become used to exploiting the illusion of quick fixes that take the complex challenges of health systems out of the headlines, whilst no doubt being aware of the magnitude of the task required to genuinely transform health services. This is why some have promoted the idea of taking health outside of politics altogether. The concept is not without merit, but there are two major barriers to it ever happening. Firstly, health and care are accountable for an ever-increasing share of public spending; as long as services such as the NHS are directly funded from taxes, no government can escape being held accountable for their performance. Secondly, if health is re-positioned, it presents an opportunity for a brighter future, and this opportunity ought to be democratized, the sooner the better.

Genuine transformation is much harder than a quick fix, but COVID-19 provides the opportunity for bold and meaningful change.

We are willing to pay more, but we must be paying for the right things

In the post-COVID-19 world, difficult choices will have to be made. Before COVID-19, British citizens were already saying that they would be willing to pay more in tax to maintain the NHS and to protect other public services. The nation's profound appreciation for those key workers putting themselves in harm's way to keep us alive and well was borne out for ten weeks through March to May 2020 when, each Thursday at 8pm, the nation stood on their doorsteps and participated in the 'clap for carers.' We care very deeply for the free-at-point-of-delivery service that keeps us alive in our time of need.

Two thirds of the British public support the idea of paying more tax, rather than reducing the level of care provided by the NHS or reducing other public services [5]. Indeed, when asked about more specific policies, more than half of the public supported increasing the basic rate of income tax by one pence in the pound, from 20 to 21 pence, to fund the NHS, and almost two-thirds supported a raise in National Insurance (a social tax) with hypothecation for the same purpose [6].

Hypothecating funds implies that there are trade-offs to be made between health, or the NHS, versus other public services, but this is a false distinction. Our collective predilection to focus on shorter-term crises, especially when we hear so regularly how stretched our front-line services are, makes things difficult because it creates competing priorities. This is reflected in further polling; when the public were asked where extra healthcare funds should go, 68% said extra funds should go to urgent care services, with 23% arguing to spend on preventative health, despite, as we are frequently reminded, an ounce of prevention being worth a pound of cure. This, too, speaks to the need to create a real alternative in the positioning of health and health systems for the future.

From importers of illnesses to exporters of health

We talk about health, and the National Health Service, but what we really mean is being ill, and what should perhaps be called the National Illness Service. It treats our illnesses and does its best to make us healthy again, which stems from its founding principles. However, among a set of additional principles introduced in 2000 was that the NHS will: 'help to keep people healthy and work to reduce health inequalities'. This acknowledges that a better system would be focused on keeping us healthy and preventing us from getting ill and needing treatment, but we cannot expect the NHS to perform this function on its own. The only way to do this is if we recognize the true role that health plays in our lives, our communities, and our economies, and acknowledge that the NHS is part of a much broader health picture.

On top of that, we need to understand that what in the past have been thought of as determinants of health—immutable, unchangeable factors that are outside our control—should really be thought of as drivers, things that can be changed if we collectively choose to do so. Those drivers of health—biomedical, social, commercial—have changed in the past and can be changed again if society is willing.

As our health has changed, our health systems have not kept pace. In this book we argue for a total health system which comprises both the wider health environment and an expanded healthcare system, because we know that healthcare itself is responsible for less than 15% of the health we experience. On top of the illness service provided by the NHS, we also need social care. While we reap the benefits of advances in healthcare and live for longer, our health begins to fail us in different ways as we age and suffer from accumulating conditions. Social care, whether in an individual's own home or an institution, is pivotal to that person living well and independently for as long as possible. Doing this well clearly reduces the demands on hospitals and primary care, yet the historical false distinction between health and social care services makes doing it so much harder. By building false boundaries and silos throughout the system, we make it more difficult to have a patient-centred system and we all, individuals, services, and nations, lose.

Putting health first needs wide-scale change and, with the complexities that keep us healthy or unhealthy, the roles of government policy and industry, the environment we live in, and the healthcare service itself, this is a major challenge. But without a change of direction, we can expect to see further modest increases in longevity mask growing ill health across societies, hampering economic prosperity and fairness. Progress in reducing some drivers of ill health will be masked by new social and commercial drivers of ill health, many symptomatic of globalization and the loosening rules-based-system that does not have at its heart the health, happiness, and prosperity of individuals, communities, and societies.

Health and health systems must be repositioned and revalued

We believe that health should be recognized as the most untapped driver of prosperity, happiness, and social mobility in the 21st century. The COVID-19 pandemic has demonstrated that health is a precious resource and should be valued as such. It has also demonstrated that viewing health as an asset, not a problem to be cured, could be a game-changer in a post-COVID-19 world.

COVID-19 gives us a pivotal moment, and choices that have been put off for years can no longer be avoided. The interdependency of our health, the economy, and wider society has become clearer than ever, and we can see that poor physical health is only one of the impacts of a complex scenario. Indirect effects on the health and wealth of the nation will also be felt in the form of increased unemployment, a worsening economy, and a rise in mental ill health and social issues arising from the unequal lived experiences of the pandemic.

Recovery will depend on promoting the health of citizens in the broadest sense, both in individuals being healthy enough to work, and also in creating health-promoting environments that maximize opportunities for all.

With that concept at the forefront, we can re-design our health system to be a complete package delivering health, quality of life, and sustainability, whilst supporting individuals to live healthy lives and remain independent for as long as possible. Putting health rather than illness first today could pay real dividends for other public services and the finances of the nation in years to come.

Repositioning and valuing health is part of a holistic vision that could unlock years of prosperity and happiness across communities and the nation by:

- reducing inequalities in education and work;
- enabling social mobility;

- rebalancing the social and physical environment to make it easy to be healthy;
- identifying shared values between industries and communities; and
- shifting healthcare systems from importers of illness to exporters of health.

As nations begin to rebuild after COVID-19, they can no longer take health for granted. If, as we propose, health becomes recognized for the asset it is and is repositioned as an opportunity rather than a burden, then at least some good would have come from this awful pandemic. Our future is in our hands and we can shape it; COVID-19 is the wake-up call to show that an aspirational future is within reach if governments and societies choose it.

In this book, we explore a range of issues that feed into the complexity of health and its function in society today, and describe our proposals for a set of new social contracts, New NHS, New Public Health, and New Shared Values, which should underpin our health and prosperity going forward. But first, we need to talk about the definition of health.

References

1. Ipsos MORI. *Veracity Index 2019*. November 2019: https://www.ipsos.com/ipsos-mori/en-uk/trust-politicians-falls-sending-them-spiralling-back-bottom-ipsos-mori-veracity-index
2. Max Roser and Esteban Ortiz-Ospina (2013). *Global Extreme Poverty*. Published online at OurWorldInData.org. Retrieved from: https://ourworldindata.org/extreme-poverty
3. NHS Digital. *Health Survey for England 2017: Adult and child overweight and obesity*. November 2019: https://files.digital.nhs.uk/EF/AB0F0C/HSE17-Adult-Child-BMI-rep-v2.pdf. Baker C. *Obesity Statistics. House of Commons Library*. August 2019. Accessed via: https://commonslibrary.parliament.uk/research-briefings/sn03336/
4. OECD. *Health at a Glance 2017*. OECD. November 2017: http://www.oecd.org/newsroom/healthier-lifestyles-and-better-health-policies-drive-life-expectancy-gains.htm
5. IPSOS Mori. NHS at 70: Public Attitudes to the health and care system. May 2018. Accessed via: https://www.ipsos.com/ipsos-mori/en-uk/nhs-70-public-attitudes-health-and-care-system
6. YouGov. A Majority of Brits now support increasing income tax to fund the NHS. July 2018, Accessed via: https://yougov.co.uk/topics/politics/articles-reports/2018/07/03/majority-brits-now-support-increasing-income-tax-f

2

Are we healthy? It's complicated

Better health is central to human happiness and well-being. Health also makes an important contribution to economic progress, as healthy populations live longer, are more productive, and save more.

World Health Organization

Introducing total health

In England, the Department of Health and Social Care spends more than 95% of its budget on the National Health Service (NHS), which, as we mentioned in Chapter 1, could better be described as the National Illness Service because health tends to be defined as what it is not, rather than an holistic state of well-being.

The World Health Organization (WHO) has a different perspective, and defines health as a state of complete physical, mental, and social well-being, and not merely the absence of disease or infirmity. Actually, they go further and say that physical and mental well-being to enable a life without limitation or restriction is a human right. But in practice, is that what we as individuals think and is that how nations act?

WHO builds on its broad definition of health with two measures, Disability Adjusted Life Years (DALYs) and Quality Adjusted Life Years (QALYs), that help to fill out the picture somewhat. DALYs are an official estimate used to capture more than just life expectancy or mortality, but also years of life lost due to ill health, disability, or death, and they are a move in the right direction for health systems trying to promote health (or lost health) and living well rather than illness or death. But one of the difficulties is that measuring years lost is challenging to calculate and does not capture the whole lived experience of a disease, as no two people will experience a particular disease in exactly the same way.

The National Institute for Health and Care Excellence (NICE) in the UK uses QALYs to assess the cost-effectiveness of drugs and interventions. It is

Whose Health Is It, Anyway? Dame Sally C. Davies and Jonathan Pearson-Stuttard, Oxford University Press (2021).
© Oxford University Press. DOI: 10.1093/oso/9780198863458.003.0002

positive that they use this measure to take quality of life into account, but currently it is only done through a single-disease lens. To truly capture what DALYs and QALYs aim for, we need a more holistic, multimorbid approach, from the perspective of both patients and health systems.

To capture the WHO definition and its wider ramifications, we are introducing the concept of 'total health'. Total health includes physical, mental, and social health, and also the underlying drivers that influence all those aspects of our lives. Health with a capital 'H', if you like. Putting the idea of total health at the forefront of some of the most critical challenges we face enables us to embrace the complexities of the modern world, and move beyond siloed thinking about individual illnesses.

What makes up our total health and our ill health has changed over time, as has the role total health plays in our lives. There has been a shift from illness threatening our longevity to poor health preventing our enjoyment of life, lowering productivity, and reducing prosperity. But governments around the world still view health through the illness lens, as a drain on resources and a barrier to longevity. We, the public, play along; we care about health, but this usually translates into caring about the service that keeps us living, not necessarily in good health, and often not intervening until it is too late.

Total health is an opportunity to embrace a new paradigm for prosperity and well-being, and to address some of the ills of society today in a holistic and meaningful manner.

In this chapter, we examine two aspects of total health: the issues inherent in how we view our health today and the role societal inequalities play in damaging health and life chances.

What does it mean to feel healthy?

Public opinion about health is quite mixed. Globally, only around half of us (56%) agree that we feel in good health, with the Indian population being the most satisfied at 70%, the US and UK following at 64% and 59% respectively. The least satisfied are the Japanese, with just 32% of the population reporting that they feel in good health [1].

Cancer, obesity, and mental ill health dominate global health discussions, and awareness of poor diet and physical inactivity as key drivers of cancer and obesity is increasing. Along with this, we tend to perceive, and want to believe, that we lead healthier lifestyles than we actually do; 48% of the world feel that they eat a healthy diet and 40% feel they get enough exercise—far higher than the reality.

Looking forward a decade, the public are not optimistic. Only 21% of British citizens think their health will be better in 10 years, with 31% feeling it will be worse. As we age, maintaining good health becomes more and more important to each of us. Feeling in control over our own health, and whether our ill health prevents us doing what we want to do, matters if we are to enjoy our own lives to the fullest, and support friends and family when they need us.

There is much more optimism about future health in emerging economies, such as India (where 66% believe their health will be better in a decade) and China (57%), perhaps tying optimism about their health to increasing wealth as both nations continue through an economic transition.

Japan has the second longest life expectancy in the world at 84.7 years, yet the most pessimistic outlook, with just 11% believing their health will be better in 10 years. Perhaps the Japanese are leading the charge, placing greater value on the quality of years lived in a state of well-being, and reflecting how health in the 21st century affects our lives, for good and bad.

Increasing life expectancy is a good thing, right?

By most traditional measures, our health has improved greatly over the past 70 years. There are more than 7.6 billion people in the world today, three times the number there were in 1950, but the total number of deaths each year is still about the same, despite this. A whole host of advances have contributed to such impressive gains, but the greatest reductions in early death risk have been in children under five years of age, through improvements in living conditions, sanitation, and access to healthcare, particularly vaccinations.

At every age, and for every decade since World War 2, the risk of each of us dying has fallen, allowing us all to live longer than ever before [2]. Globally, the average person can now expect to live for almost 70 years—some 22 years more than in 1950. And every country has seen big improvements in life expectancy; in Ethiopia it was 33.3 years in 1950, increasing to 61.6 years today, whilst a person born in the UK can now expect to live to 80.4 years, 12 years more than in 1950.

These improvements have not been continuous though, and natural disasters, conflicts, and economic shocks, such as the Great Leap Forward in China from 1958 to 1962, have all taken their toll. Epidemics of infectious diseases such as HIV/AIDS have halted, and even reversed, progress in some places, whilst health systems have been slow to react and combat unforeseen events. We have been here before, and COVID-19 reminds us that we will inevitably face other challenges to longevity, including pandemics, in the future.

Nor have the impressive improvements in longevity been matched by living in good health; today we are living a greater portion of our lives in poor health. In the UK, for example, life expectancy in 2017 was 79.6 years for men and 83.2 years for women, however, the last 16 and 19 years, respectively, are lived in poor health (see Fig. 2.1) [3]. Given that British men can retire in their mid-60s, they can expect to spend a lot of their retirement in ill health, unable to either fully enjoy their new-found freedom or to support other family members as they may wish, and these limitations often affect their mental and social health. A woman in the most deprived 30% retiring at 60 years of age will spend the vast majority of the rest of her life living in ill health.

This trend of unexpected consequences associated with improvements in life expectancy is true for many specific diseases, too. Our risk of dying from conditions such as diabetes has reduced dramatically, but the effects of this disease on day-to-day lives are worsening. Those in Germany with diabetes have seen modest increases in life expectancy over the past 15 years, but the proportion of their lives lived with diabetes and its health effects has increased by more than 10%, much more than the relative increase in life expectancy [4].

The causes of ill health have changed

Perversely, living longer means we are at risk of developing a wider range of problems, and more of them. The improvement in life expectancy over the last 70 years has been accompanied by a shift in the conditions and diseases that shape our ill health, from predominantly infectious diseases to non-communicable diseases (NCDs, also referred to as non-infectious diseases). The largest contributors to this shift, often referred to as the 'epidemiological transition', have been dramatic declines in deaths due to infectious diseases along with a rise in vascular diseases (such as heart disease and stroke), and, more recently, diabetes and obesity.

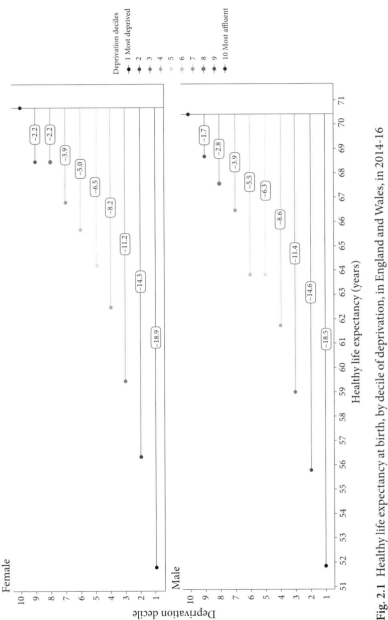

Fig. 2.1 Healthy life expectancy at birth, by decile of deprivation, in England and Wales, in 2014–16

Reproduced from Davies SC, Annual Report of the Chief Medical Officer, 2018. Health 2040 – Better Health Within Reach, Copyright (2018), Department of Health and Social Care. Reproduced under the Open Government Licence v3.0. Original source: data from Office for National Statistics statistical bulletin, Health state life expectancies by national deprivation deciles, England and Wales: 2014 to 2016, Copyright (2018), Office for National Statistics.

Infectious diseases of decades ago were generally short term and intense, tend to strike in younger years, and require treatments (for instance antibiotics) that, typically, lead to a full recovery. Living through infections then means we are vulnerable to vascular diseases, which tend to strike at a later age. Vascular diseases such as ischaemic heart disease are often life-long, risk being managed rather than removed, and result in an increased risk of premature death from several causes.

Cancers generally come into the equation later in life, and dementia at a later age still. That dementia became the leading cause of death in the UK in 2018 speaks to our success in living longer—we are dying from diseases that affect us later in life—but this, once again, masks the accumulation of ill health with which we are living.

A more recent transition has been in the nature of long-term conditions experienced. As death rates from vascular diseases have declined since the 1980s thanks to lower rates of smoking and better treatments, diabetes and obesity have increased. These conditions bring with them an increased risk of early death, but perhaps more than that, they also bring a much greater risk of acquiring several other conditions, each with their own substantive impacts on daily ill health.

The epidemiological transition has been experienced at a different pace around the world. High-income western countries completed the transition in the mid-to-late 20th century, whilst many low- and middle-income countries are in the midst of this transition now, often facing the challenge of coping with major infectious diseases, such as HIV and TB, and the emerging tide of NCDs at the same time.

The drivers of health in a society where infectious diseases dominate the burden of ill health have predominantly been due to an environment of insufficiency; lack of things like safe drinking water, good sanitation, and adequate housing, factors that reflect a society at the earlier stages of economic development. In contrast, many of the drivers of NCD ill health are often described as a state of excess; too much unhealthy, high-calorie food, too much alcohol, too much sedentary time, too much pollution, and smoking.

The reality, of course, is more complex and nuanced, since our total health is a combination of genetic, physiological, behavioural, and environmental risks. These risks combine and amplify each other, for instance genetic mutations that make an individual crave yet more food after a substantial meal are compounded if that person lives in an obesogenic environment, where calorie-rich food is readily available and cheap. Sedentary lifestyles lead to a weakened physiological state, but so does living in a crowded urban environment where there is little opportunity to exercise outside. Social media affects those who use it to compare themselves unfavourably with others, influencing their mental health detrimentally, but it can also be a force for good if harnessed in the right way.

So the dichotomy of classifying diseases as infectious or non-infectious and the idea of an epidemiological transition is to some extent artificial, and has become less meaningful and useful for patients and health services. We now know that several so-called NCDs are in fact caused by infectious diseases; hepatitis C (a viral infection) is the leading cause of liver cancer, which is on the rise globally, and human papillomavirus (HPV) is responsible for around 70% of all cervical cancers, a leading cause of death in young women.

Similarly, the traditional view that infections are short term and NCDs longer term, with implications for how we prevent and treat them, is outdated in many cases. In the 1980s, a diagnosis with HIV meant a life expectancy of just a few months coloured by ill health. Today, those with HIV have a near-normal life expectancy and, in most cases, their diagnosed condition has little bearing on their day-to-day life [5].

More of us are living with multiple morbidities

We have been very successful in reducing our risk of dying prematurely, but much less successful at preventing or curing the diseases our later years bring. Worse still, these diseases and health conditions gradually accumulate as we age.

Living with more than one chronic condition—'multimorbidity'—is now the norm in the UK (see Fig. 2.2). Around 10% of the UK population have at least four long-term conditions, a statistic forecast to nearly double by 2035 [6]. The two biggest drivers of multimorbidity—age and relative deprivation—are also forecast to increase over the next 15 years. We've already seen how advancing age makes us more susceptible to becoming less healthy, but we also find that multimorbidity is 20% more prevalent in the poorest communities, and those same groups are shockingly 90% more likely to have 10 or more functional limitations as they age.

People living with conditions such as diabetes and obesity are often typical of those living with multimorbidity. Diabetes and obesity increase the risk of getting many other conditions—including several common cancers, heart disease, strokes, liver disease, back pain, and depression and anxiety. Extreme complications of diabetes include amputation and blindness.

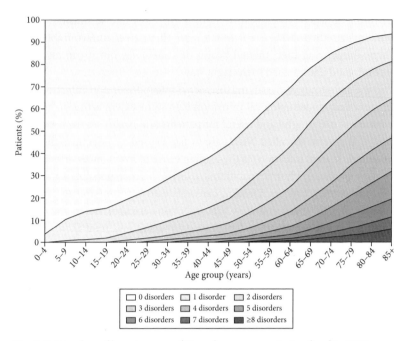

Fig. 2.2 Number of long term conditions by age group in Scotland in 2012

Reproduced from Davies SC, Annual Report of the Chief Medical Officer, 2018. Health
2040 – Better Health Within Reach, Copyright (2018), Department of Health and Social Care.
Reproduced under the Open Government Licence v3.0. Original source: Reproduced from
Lancet, 380(9836), Barnett K, Mercer SW, Norbury M, et al., Epidemiology of multimorbidity
and implications for health care, research, and medical education: a cross-sectional study,
pp. 37–43, Copyright (2012), with permission from Elsevier Ltd.

Many of the most common conditions driving multimorbidity have shared
drivers; poor diet, excess alcohol consumption, smoking, physical inactivity,
and air pollution. These five risk factors, all of which are preventable, account
for more than 50% of all ill health in the UK. So tackling multimorbidity is
not just about immediate health-related interventions but goes much wider
than that. Working on all these drivers simultaneously would pay dividends
for employers, the national economy, the NHS, and individuals.

Health haves and have-nots

We may be in this together, but that doesn't mean we are in this
equally.

Paul Johnson, Director, Institute for Fiscal Studies

Progress in longevity has not been felt equally, either between countries or within them; the nature of our ill health may have changed, but the inequalities are entrenched. The seminal UK Whitehall study in 1991 compellingly concluded that a big inverse association exists between social class and the risk of death from a wide range of common diseases. Simply put, the lower the social class of an individual, the higher their risk of death.

In the UK, for example, in 2000, a woman in the most deprived 10% of the population could expect to live six years less than a woman from the least deprived 10%. By 2016, this gap had increased to eight years. The gap in life expectancy worsened in men over this period too—from nine to ten years (see Fig. 2.3).

Death rates from coronary heart disease have declined by as much as 70% over the past three decades, making a big contribution to the increases in life expectancy. Half of this improvement is credited to improvement in factors such as smoking. But since smoking prevalence is twice as high in the most deprived groups compared to the most affluent, it is not surprising that these improvements have not been felt equally [7].

The gap in years lived in good health as we age (healthy life expectancy) between different groups in UK society is worse still—almost double that of life expectancy as we saw in Fig. 2.1. Women from the most deprived 10% in the UK can expect to live just 51.8 years in good health, some 19.9 years less than the least deprived 10%; the gap for men is marginally less (18.5 years). Living in poor health from the age of 52 is not just miserable for the individual and their family, it also holds back the prosperity of local communities and the nation as a whole; a healthier nation is a wealthier one, for everybody.

These deteriorating health states seem to be forging new inequalities. Not only are those with diabetes or obesity at increased risk of contracting a host of other conditions, but they are also likely to suffer from worse educational outcomes and thus worse job opportunities. At every turn, these conditions get bleaker.

Health, education, and work interact to shape our life chances

The idea that our own health is an important contributor to our economic outlook, life chances, and human capital is logical and has been around for some time. Today, we are learning more about the complex relationships

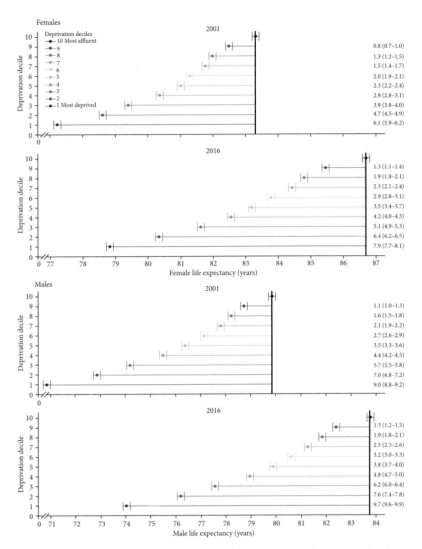

Fig. 2.3 Life expectancy at birth, by decile of deprivation, and sex, in England, in 2001 and 2016

Reproduced from Davies SC, Annual Report of the Chief Medical Officer, 2018. Health 2040 – Better Health Within Reach, Copyright (2018), Department of Health and Social Care. Reproduced under the Open Government Licence v3.0. Original source: Reproduced from Lancet Public Health, 3(12), Bennett JE, Pearson-Stuttard J, Kontis V, et al., Contributions of diseases and injuries to widening life expectancy inequalities in England from 2001 to 2016: a population-based analysis of vital registration data, pp. E586-E597, Copyright (2018), Elsevier Ltd. Reproduced under the Creative Commons Attribution 4.0 International License (CC BY 4.0) linking health and prosperity and how this affects communities and whole nations.

We know that healthier people generally lead happier and more economically productive lives; better income and factors associated with better income are well-established social drivers of our health. In health, we can study at school and put our best foot forward at work, just as the reverse is true. Health is now a better predictor of economic attainment and job prospects than education.

In Chapter 2 of the 2018 Annual Report of the Chief Medical Officer, Paul Johnson and colleagues from the Institute for Fiscal Studies (IFS) discussed how employment is a key mediator in the relationship between health and overall prosperity [8]. They found a negative cycle of poor health clustering with poor employment opportunities and low economic productivity, with each of these factors negatively reinforcing the others. This is borne out by the statistics, which demonstrate that poor health is a barrier to secure, meaningful employment; pre-COVID-19, 70% of those with long-term conditions were in work compared with 88% of those without (see Fig. 2.4) [9]. Long-term conditions, meanwhile, are more prevalent in more deprived areas, adding further barriers to social mobility.

This is not just confined to physical illness. Over the past 20 years in the UK we have seen a 65% increase in mental ill health as a cause of incapacity benefit claim [9]. This is now a leading cause of disability across the world, and cruelly, tends to affect us at younger ages than many physical conditions, yet be persistent and often lifelong. This exerts a huge negative influence on shaping our outlook and is all too often overlooked and underfunded by governments and employers.

Inequality matters to those experiencing it and to society more widely. A child who grows up in one of the most deprived neighbourhoods in England is twice as likely to be obese when they start and finish primary school as a child growing up in the least deprived neighbourhood. This disadvantage holds these children back throughout life, affecting their learning and job opportunities. Those with the lowest levels of education have about twice the likelihood of being out of work compared with those with higher levels of education. Being in good health is also pivotal in this relationship. Those with the same level of education, but in good health, have a much higher chance of securing stable employment. Low levels of education and poor health impact the chances of people of getting into employment and then staying in work.

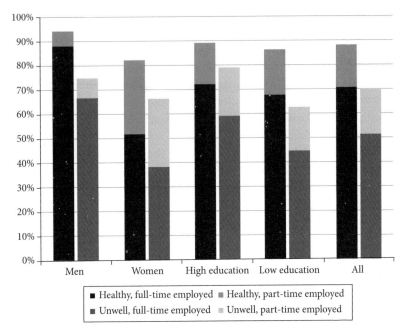

Fig. 2.4 Employment status of 25- to 54-year-olds with and without a longstanding illness, 2016–17, Great Britain

Reproduced from Davies SC, Annual Report of the Chief Medical Officer, 2018. Health 2040 – Better Health Within Reach, Copyright (2018), Department of Health and Social Care. Reproduced under the Open Government Licence v3.0. Original source: Reproduced from Cribb J, Keiller AN, Waters T, Living standards, poverty and inequality in the UK: 2018, Copyright (2018), with permission from The Institute for Fiscal Studies.

This disadvantage is relentless; these same children from our most deprived neighbourhoods will have been 17 times more likely to have been exposed to smoking during pregnancy, and have a higher risk of early death from a number of conditions. Our most deprived communities are also more likely to experience mental ill health, in turn reducing their likelihood of stable and meaningful employment.

Historically, being in work was the surest way out of poverty and a platform for social mobility within communities. This alone, however, is no longer enough: 50% of adults living in relative poverty in the UK are in fact in working households, a tragic statistic. This is even more concerning when we learn that 70% of children in poverty are in working households [10]. Do we really need the UN Convention on the Rights of the Child to tell us that every child has a right to be born into a world that promotes, rather than harms, their health, with a healthy environment providing a fair grounding for social mobility? [11]

Education, alongside work, has long been a key policy target for improving prosperity and reducing the gap in opportunities across and within communities. However, improvements in the three key traits of health, education, and employment are not randomly distributed across the country, but instead cluster together. There are areas where they are all on the up, pushing local communities to brighter futures, and other areas where the reverse is true.

In Blackpool, north-west England, for example, unemployment (claimant) rates are some of the highest in the country, at 13% in 2018, compared with just 4% in Woking, south-east England. This same area suffers the highest smoking-in-pregnancy rates in the country at 28%, whereas it is just 2% in Woking [12]. The reasons women continue to smoke during pregnancy are complex and highly personal, so the usual one-size-fits-all approach to this problem has, unsurprisingly, widened rather than closed the inequality gap. This is then reflected in persistent unfairness throughout life, leading to the life-expectancy gaps in women and men of 8 and 10 years, respectively. The vicious cycle of poor health, low educational attainment, and precarious employment continues.

COVID-19 shines an unforgiving light on health inequalities

COVID-19 has illustrated the extremes of how the prospects of health, education, and work cluster together in the haves and the have nots. Just three months into the pandemic, the unequal effects of the virus and policy responses such as lockdown were already clear.

The poorest in society have been more at risk of catching the virus and more likely to die from it. Obesity increases the risk of dying from COVID by around 40%, and obesity rates are twice as high in deprived neighbourhoods compared with the most affluent; calorie-rich take-away shops are more dense in these areas, too [13]. Those living in deprived communities are also more likely to suffer from other underlying health conditions that make them more susceptible to the virus.

As schools across the UK and much of Europe closed, substituting the learning experience in a home environment was much easier for some than others. Those in higher-income households were around 30% more likely to report that their secondary schools provided online classes and access to online interaction with teachers compared with the poorest 20% of households. Similarly, those same children from higher-income families reported 30% more time spent on home learning than children from poorer families [14]. We know the home environment is socially patterned too, with over-crowded homes and the lack of outdoor space also contributing to the lockdown period widening inequalities in education.

During the COVID-19 lockdown, employment levels were hit dramatically. Younger adults were disproportionately affected, as were the lowest earners [15]. Those in the bottom 10% of earners were seven times more likely to work in sectors that closed during lockdown compared to the top earners.

In April 2020, the number of people claiming unemployment benefit shot up to more than 2 million, around 5.8% of the population. For comparison, this figure never breached 5% after the 2008 recession. When we add to this that one in four of the UK workforce, some 7.5 million people, were on furlough—a scheme whereby the Government covered 80% of an employee's salary up to £2,500 per month—unemployment rates are clearly going to get worse before they get better.

For those for whom work continued during lockdown, the lowest paid were most likely to be key workers, in occupations that increased the risk of catching the virus, whether through travelling to work, or due to the nature of their job. In May 2020, Transport for London announced an independent review into the factors behind the COVID-19 deaths of 29 bus drivers and 4 other transport staff in London [16].

Joblessness will affect the health of people and communities today and in the coming months and years. Estimates suggest that, if unemployment levels reach those experienced after the 2008 crisis, this will lead to 900,000 more working age people suffering from chronic health conditions, and the numbers of those with mental ill health will rise by 500,000 [17]. Once the acute phase of the pandemic has passed, these more stubborn ill health patterns will hold communities, companies, and the nation back as we try to rebuild.

The adverse effects of COVID-19 on education and employment themselves worsen the outlook for total health, with the most vulnerable most heavily hit once more. On top of this, the direct health effects of COVID-19 have already exacerbated unfairness in health outcomes. Those from the most deprived 20% have been twice as likely to die from the virus than those from the most affluent 20% [18]. Black African men have been nearly four times more likely to die than the male population average, with many Black, Asian and Minority Ethnic (BAME) groups at much higher risk, whether patients or health and care staff [19].

On top of this, COVID-19 already looks set to have long-term effects on our health. It may make us more susceptible to other infectious diseases or worsen the trajectories of existing chronic conditions, and it is expected to have an effect on mental and social health, particularly in patients who need a long period of rehabilitation before they can return to normal life.

It had become clear before the pandemic how interlinked education, work, and health are in the life prospects of individuals, their communities, and whole nations. COVID-19 will widen the gap in society for generations, unless we think and act differently.

This all speaks to the need for a change in how we value health.

Total health

Given the staggering 19-year gap in years of life lived in good health between the most and least deprived 10% in England today, the clear inequalities in the impact of COVID-19 on different groups in society, and the growing understanding of the multifarious factors influencing what it means to be healthy, we need a new approach to our health.

Living well for longer matters to us all, but that does not mean simply treating us when we become ill; it also means preventing the onset of disease, enabling us to live well and independently with long-term conditions, and encompassing all the elements that contribute to our total health, not just those directly related to illness.

The total health approach is less focused on which organ might be failing at a given rate, or which hospital specialist is most suited for each of our many chronic conditions; instead, it makes health personal, respects the lived experience, and removes as many barriers as possible so that we each have a platform for a happy and healthy day-to-day life.

In the next chapter, we ask to what extent our current health system is built for this new approach, and how we should start to think about a system for the future that is built on total health, not just healthcare.

References

1. IPSOS Global Advisors. *Global views on healthcare*. 2018: https://www.ipsos.com/ sites/default/files/ct/news/documents/2018-07/global-views-on-healthcare-2018-ipsos-global-advisor.pdf

2. GBD 2017 Mortality Collaborators. Global, regional, and national age-sex-specific mortality and life expectancy, 1950–2017: a systematic analysis for the Global Burden of Disease Study 2017. *The* Lancet 2018; 392:1684–735: https://www.thelancet.com/pdfs/journals/lancet/PIIS0140-6736(18)31891-9.pdf
3. Public Health England. *Health profile for England:2018*. September 2018: https://www.gov.uk/government/publications/health-profile-for-england-2018
4. Muschik D, Tetzlaff J, Lange K, Epping J, Eberhard S, Geyer S. Change in life expectancy with type 2 diabetes: a study using claims data from lower Saxony, Germany. *Population Health Metrics*. 2017;15(1):5
5. Antiretroviral Therapy Cohort Collaboration. Survival of HIV-positive patients starting antiretroviral therapy between 1996 and 2013: a collaborative analysis of cohort studies. *The* Lancet HIV. 2017;4(8):e349–e56. doi:10.1016/S2352-3018(17)30066-8: https://www.nhs.uk/news/mental-health/life-expectancy-for-people-with-hiv-now-near-normal/
6. Kingston A, Robinson L, Booth H, Knapp M, Jagger C. Projections of multimorbidity in the older population in England to 2035: estimates from the Population Ageing and Care Simulation (PACSim) model. *Age and Ageing*. 2018;47(3):374–80.
7. Action on Smoking and Health. *Health inequalities and smoking*. September 2019: https://ash.org.uk/wp-content/uploads/2019/09/ASH-Briefing_Health-Inequalities.pdf
8. Davies S. *Annual Report of the Chief Medical Officer, 2018, Health 2040–Better Health Within Reach*. London: Department of Health and Social Care, 2018.
9. Emmerson C, Joyce R, Sturrock D. Working-age Incapacity and disability benefit. In: Emmerson C, Johnson P, Joyce R, (eds.), *IFS Green Budget 2017*. February 2017.
10. Department for Work and Pensions. *Households below average income: 1994/95—2017/18*. March 2019: https://www.gov.uk/government/statistics/households-below-average-income-199495-to-201718
11. Mytton OT, Fenton-Glynn C, Pawson E, Viner RM, Davies SC. Protecting children's rights: why governments must be bold to tackle childhood obesity. *The* Lancet. 2019;394(10207):1393–95. doi:10.1016/S0140-6736(19)32274-3
12. NHS Digital. Statistics on women's smoking status at time of delivery, England—Quarter 4, 2016–17. NHS Digital. 2017.
13. Office for National Statistics. National Child Measurement Programme, England 2017/18 school year. NHS Digital. 2018: https://files.digital.nhs.uk/9F/22AF4D/nati-chil-meas-prog-eng-2017-2018-rep.pdf
14. Andrew A, Cattan S, Costa-Dias M, et al. Learning during the lockdown: real-time data on children's experiences during home learning. *IFS Briefing Note BN288*. May 2020.
15. Banks J, Karjalainen H, Propper C. Recessions and health: The long-term health consequences of responses to coronavirus. *IFS Briefing Note BN281*. April 2020.
16. Transport for London. Review into coronavirus infections and deaths among bus workers. 21 May 2020: https://tfl.gov.uk/info-for/media/press-releases/2020/may/review-into-coronavirus-infections-and-deaths-among-bus-workers

17. Janke K, Lee K, Propper C, et al. Macroeconomic conditions and health in Britain: aggregation, dynamics and local area heterogeneity. Centre for Economic Policy Research (CEPR), *Discussion Paper DP14507*. April 2020.
18. Office for National Statistics. Deaths involving COVID-19 by local area and socioeconomic deprivation: deaths occurring between 1 March and 31 May 2020. June 2020: https://www.ons.gov.uk/peoplepopulationandcommunity/birthsdeathsandmarriages/deaths/bulletins/deathsinvolvingcovid19bylocalareasanddeprivation/deathsoccurringbetween1marchand31may2020
19. Office for National Statistics. Coronavirus (COVID-19) related deaths by ethnic group, England and Wales: 2 March 2020 to 10 April 2020. May 2020: https://www.ons.gov.uk/peoplepopulationandcommunity/birthsdeathsandmarriages/deaths/articles/coronavirusrelateddeathsbyethnicgroupenglandandwales/2march2020to10april2020

3

Is our health system ready for the future?

The National Health Service (NHS) is a source of deep pride to British citizens because of the enduring principles it was founded upon—universal access to healthcare for all, free at the point of use. The ability to receive often lifesaving care without fear or favour, at a time when we are at our most vulnerable, is deeply emotive. Essentially, the NHS is a form of national health insurance funded out of taxation for the benefit of all, protecting those who become ill. The British people look at other systems, including the USA, and see our system as fundamental to a progressive society. We hear with horror of patients' wallets being checked before treatment can begin, or astronomical hospital bills when being discharged after going through a life-changing disaster.

> *The NHS is the closest thing most British people have to a religion.*
>
> Nigel Lawson

The NHS matters even more locally, as an anchor institution in our communities. Yes, it keeps us alive and is there without any judgement or prejudice in our hour of need, but it is also the largest employer (both direct and indirect) in many regions and a big contributor to local economic activity. In the early weeks of COVID-19 the lockdown message was to 'stay at home, protect the NHS, save lives'—apparently valuing the NHS for more than just the lives it saves.

In the UK, health and the NHS are consistently priorities for voters in general elections. In the general election in 2017, health was more important than Brexit for voters when they were asked about local priorities and what would influence their voting decision. When voters were asked to consider the national situation, they put Brexit above health—but Brexit still had a smaller influence than health on how they would actually vote in their constituency [1].

Launched in July 1948, the NHS was designed in the post-World War 2 period, when treating acute infections and discharging patients back into the community were its primary objectives. We clearly still depend

Whose Health Is It, Anyway? Dame Sally C. Davies and Jonathan Pearson-Stuttard, Oxford University Press (2021).
© Oxford University Press. DOI: 10.1093/oso/9780198863458.003.0003

on that service, but, as we have seen, the health scenario of the population has changed dramatically, and so has our satisfaction with the services the NHS provides. In 2018, public satisfaction with the NHS had fallen to just 53%. The primary reasons for dissatisfaction were 'long waiting times, staff shortages, lack of funding and money being wasted' [2].

This chapter looks at how we understand our health system now, and some of the issues we must start to address. We also explore how we envisage a future that, after the first wave of the COVID-19 pandemic, looks very different from a future we might have predicted six months ago. The future is necessarily a moving target, but we have to imagine it if we are to face the challenges it will inevitably bring.

The NHS is not the only ingredient in our health system

Our health system is not just the NHS. The NHS is the healthcare part of the entire ecosystem that affects our health, which encompasses not only treating our illnesses, but also helping us to live healthier lives for longer. What we refer to as the 'health ecosystem' is actually made up of three elements: NHS and social care; public health; and the world around us—the wider health environment—which includes global industry, government, commerce, and a number of other external factors that influence the world we live in. Health, good health, and lack of illness all have a number of drivers that interact, and a holistic health system for total health takes account of all of these.

Social care is fundamental to living well in older age. Delivered properly, accepting that health is personal to each of us as we age, it can help minimize costs and can bring huge relief and better quality of life to individuals and their families. Delivered badly, not coordinated with health services, and not designed around the individual, it is costly and rarely leads to healthy communities.

Accounting for £20bn of annual expenditure, social care has been a Cinderella service for too long in the UK, with a workforce greatly undervalued for the key role they play in lives and communities. Just one in four people in the UK are satisfied with the social care service, half of the number that are satisfied with the NHS itself. Before COVID-19 hit, the British public were pessimistic about the future of social care, with over 50% of the UK population fearing that services would deteriorate over the next 12 months [3]. COVID-19 will only have entrenched this pessimism further.

During the first phase of COVID-19, deaths in care homes were higher than in any other setting compared to normal times. At the peak of the first wave, deaths in hospitals were up by nearly 90%, but up by 220% in care homes [4]. Care homes, despite the high density of vulnerable individuals, were not prioritized for early COVID-19 testing and personal protective equipment (PPE) hence in April 2020, with more than 18,000 excess deaths across care homes, less than half of these were formally recorded as related to COVID-19.

This wave of excess deaths highlighted the lack of protection and systematic planning across social care compared to the NHS, and left many of our most vulnerable citizens—the elderly with excess health risks and the care workforce, many with precarious social circumstances—at risk.

Illness is costly

Our much-loved NHS accounts for a growing share of government spending and barely keeping its head above water. Many NHS trusts were already in deficit before the pandemic, and coping with COVID-19 stretched resources to the limit. The lockdown message was badged to 'save our NHS' as well as to 'save lives' because the threat to a stretched system was so serious.

The UK health budget today is around £134 billion, which accounts for 30% of all public sector spending in the UK (see Fig. 3.1). This compares to £84 billion spent on education, £37 billion on defence, and is second only to social security (£213 billion). The health budget has increased substantially over the past 60 years in terms of absolute amount, a 10-fold increase, and also as a share of government public sector spend, being just 11.2% in 1956.

This level of spending on health is expected to continue its upwards trend. Current projections suggest that, by 2050, the annual health budget will need to rise to £250 billion, 40% of all public sector spend.

Why the increase? Two over-arching reasons for our discussion: ageing populations and the fact that longer life expectancy means more years lived in ill health rather than living well; and continued medical advances and new technologies that raise the costs of treatments.

We expect the over-85 age group in the UK to double from two to four million people over the next 20 years. Each 85-year-old costs our health system more than double that of a 65-year-old, and some five times the cost of a 30-year-old. Older age groups tend to present with several conditions rather

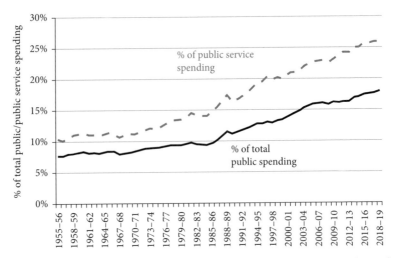

Fig. 3.1 UK public spending as a share of total public spending and as a share of public service spending

Reproduced from Stoye G, Zaranko B, UK health spending, Copyright (2019), with permission from The Institute for Fiscal Studies.

than just one, and these multimorbidities add to the complexities and costs of caring for them.

New treatments for diseases like cancer do not come cheap, and, whilst the National Institute for Health and Care Excellence (NICE) tries to keep things fair, some drugs are considered too expensive for universal use. Advances in precision medicine mean that longer lives are also on the horizon for those with rare diseases, but therapies such as the new drug Orkambi for sufferers of cystic fibrosis, an inherited disease that affects some 10,500 people in the UK, are hugely expensive.

If we continue with our current model, healthcare systems will continue to cost more and it is not unreasonable to think that rationing of certain services may increase. We have already seen the existence of a postcode lottery for women seeking IVF treatment, with the unlucky ones being unable to access the recommended three cycles, despite this being NICE guidance. Only 13% of commissioners offer the full three cycles [5].

The costs of ill health do not stop at our health and care services. Health-related benefits for those unable to work due to ill health account for £16 billion, and disability benefits cost a further £10 billion [6]. In normal (pre-COVID-19) times, this means that ill health costs the UK around £200 billion each year—more than one in every three pounds of public services spend. Alarmingly, as the healthcare system swallows up more and more funding, it is reasonable to expect that the budgets for other key public services—education, welfare, and housing—will begin to reduce, even though all of these are also key to total health and happiness.

As we have aged and accumulated more and more complex chronic health conditions, the health and care services have not kept pace. Nor have they evolved to match our health needs. Instead they continue to use a single-illness model, which does not work well for patients and is expensive for the payer. As we age and our health needs change, our demands and expectations change too.

What does the future hold for our health?

There are two kinds of forecasters: those who don't know, and those who don't know they don't know.

John Kenneth Galbraith, economist

The way that we interact with and receive healthcare today, and the way we organize and incentivize research, guidelines, and innovations, reflect our decades-old illness and treatment model. We already know that this model will not work in the future, but how do we predict what our health system will need in a rapidly changing world? Making forecasts and projections can be a dangerous pastime, but how we look at the future matters. To plan health and other public services that will meet our needs and be affordable, we need to understand what is happening today, and make careful, considered projections of how things may and could look in years to come.

But forecasts have inherent limitations—after all, we cannot know the future—and can be used for purposes far beyond their intention, creating a wary public and a polarized decision-making system when the reality is more nuanced. 'Project fear' is a term that has gained traction in the UK over the last decade, specifically relating to two referenda—Scottish Independence in 2014 and EU membership (Brexit) in 2016. Project fear, in the instance of the EU referendum, was the name given to the (largely) economic forecasts of the incumbent government under two scenarios: the status quo, continued membership; and leaving the EU. Those behind Project fear were accused of carefully selecting key messages that best served their purposes, and this raised two key issues that fuelled passionate debate on both sides.

Firstly, as with all forecasts, assumptions must be made: will recent trends continue? How quickly will a period of adjustment last? Such assumptions are made regularly in forecasting, whether for governments, businesses, or others. Assumptions enable us to look at plausible future scenarios as just one information point to inform any given decision, whilst understanding the limitations. But in the instances mentioned above, which embodied such emotive and political issues, aspects of the forecast, whether the worst-case scenario or an assumption used to discredit the validity of the forecasts themselves, were leveraged to create fear, distrust, and distain in equal measure.

Secondly, a weather forecast can be checked against subsequent reality to see how accurate it was, but we cannot do the same with forecasts that rely on estimates of future scenarios. This is because we cannot know what might have happened had we decided to follow a different one of the perhaps many options that the forecasts hypothesized. As world events rarely play out just as expected, misuse of forecasts can reduce their value in the eyes of voters or stakeholders and contribute to a degradation of trust more broadly.

Nevertheless, looking to the future and mapping what the world might look like remains a useful tool, and one we must use to the best of our abilities. In health, to be on the front foot with general and pre-emptive prevention and treatment, we need to understand how the future might unfold and how much that might vary under plausible scenarios.

Forecasts and impact analysis work were brought to the fore during COVID-19 because a huge number of complex decisions had to be made on a daily, and almost hourly, basis. Modelling from many groups informed government policies around the world, helping to forecast how many cases a country might see over a given period and what that might mean for health services and the economy. Modelling was pivotal to help with the 'what if' questions; if we enter lockdown, will we protect the NHS enough so it can treat each patient effectively without leaving patients to die because there are not enough beds or ventilators? What about opening the economy back up? In an uncertain time, modelling can provide estimates and comparisons.

One of the key benefits of using scenario planning often cited is the collaborative approach, bringing together teams across an organization, or across a whole government as in the case of COVID-19, to consider how potential changes over a range of sectors could affect future planning from the perspective of all stakeholders.

Each input to any such model has a range of uncertainties around it, even more so with something as extreme as COVID-19, which in turn creates an even larger level of uncertainty in the ultimate conclusions. This does not mean models are useless, far from it. Instead, as COVID-19 has demonstrated, they are a tool to help inform the choices that must be made by politicians, safe in the knowledge that nothing is certain.

Our future health is not a foregone conclusion, ill health is not inevitable. The conditions behind differing health scenarios are choices and reflect a society's priorities, even if we feel powerless in pushing for change.

How do we understand total health to plan for the future?

In order to plan for the healthcare system that we will need in the future, we have to understand the underlying drivers of health, which are multiple, interrelated, and not just the obvious ones, such as the prevalence of a particular disease or condition. For instance, we know that the world's population is growing and ageing. Global forecasts suggest age- and lifestyle-related chronic diseases will continue to rise to 2040 (see Fig. 3.2). We expect this to continue in the UK, with the ratio of working age to retirement age population expected to increase from 0.27 in 2016 to 0.40 in 2040. This will have huge implications for health and care systems. We also expect diabetes and obesity to continue to dominate the burden of ill health on individual lives, health systems, and economies, and the growing prevalence of conditions such as dementia to increase the complexity of the nation's health and its dependency on a range of services.

But what and who influences and determines our health and so should be incorporated into modelling and forecasting is even broader than this. Those working in the field of public health and health more broadly refer to the 'determinants' of health, factors that play a role in our health today and in the future. However, the term determinants appears to suggest that these factors are immutable, impossible—or almost impossible—to change. This is not the case. For instance, we have seen in the past how improved sanitation has dramatically reduced childhood mortality, and how HIV/AIDS, a disease once thought untreatable, has become a lifelong condition rather than a death sentence. More recently, during the COVID-19 lockdown in April 2020, unprecedented shifts in traffic patterns drastically reduced emissions; so much so that there were an estimated 1,700 fewer pollution-related deaths that month alone [7]. We therefore, prefer 'drivers' to 'determinants' when talking about what and who influence our total health.

Looking ahead, incidence of age- and lifestyle-related diseases is expected to rise while many infectious diseases could decrease significantly.

Global baseline disease burden forecast

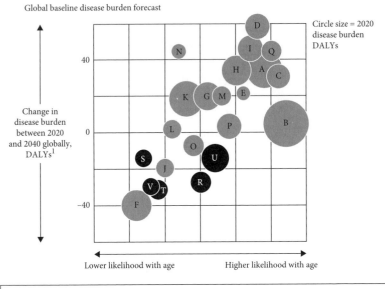

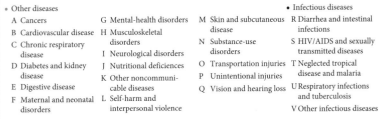

¹DALY = disability-adjusted life year.

Fig. 3.2 Global burden of chronic diseases in 2020 and forecast change in burden by 2040

In order to incorporate these drivers into our understanding of total health to create a better health system for the future, we need to understand how they combine and interact to influence the health of the individual and the health of the population in general. In 1991, Göran Dahlgren and Margaret Whitehead developed a rainbow model to explore the relationships between an individual and the different factors that impact their health (see Fig. 3.3) [8]. The model has three layers: general socio-economic, cultural, and environmental

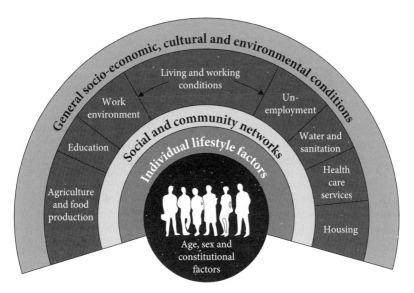

Fig. 3.3 The Dahlgren and Whitehead rainbow model of the determinants of health

Reproduced from Dahlgren G, Whitehead M (1993). Tackling inequalities in health: what can we learn from what has been tried? Working paper prepared for The King's Fund International Seminar on Tackling Inequalities in Health, September 1993, Ditchley Park, Oxfordshire. London: The King's Fund. Accessible in: Dahlgren G, Whitehead M (2007). European strategies for tackling social inequities in health: Levelling up Part 2. Copenhagen: WHO Regional office for Europe.

conditions (which includes living and working conditions, and factors such as sanitation and housing); social community networks; and individual lifestyle factors. At the centre is the individual, for whom age, sex, and constitutional factors (such as hereditary conditions) come into play. Other classifications of health determinants differ in that they try to include the extent of the influence that each factor has, perhaps attributing 30% to health behaviours, 10% to the physical environment, 10% to our genes and biology. There are though, two consistencies; the conditions in which we are born, live, and work have a substantial effect upon our health and risk of dying prematurely, and healthcare itself accounts for as little as 10% of what constitutes our health.

Pace layers—taking account of change

It is all very well having a model of the drivers of total health that incorporates several different layers of influencing factors, but a key element missing from frameworks such as Dahlgren and Whitehead's rainbow model is an understanding of how the layers interact and change. Each layer or factor is not discrete and independent, but is influenced directly by the layers on either side and indirectly by others. Understanding how the layers interact and impact on each other is essential because any changes in one layer will have knock-on effects on others. We must ensure that those ripple effects are beneficial rather than the source of unintended negative consequences.

But change is not always easy to control. We all have a sense that change is about the only thing you can count on these days. That, and the rate of change, which just keeps getting faster and more intense by the day. And there is a good reason we feel that, because quite often it is true. Take technology, for example. Driven especially by the remarkable inventions and innovations of the digital world, there are few parts of our lives that have not been completely upended and reshaped by technology. The way we connect, communicate (another Zoom call, anyone?), learn, earn, shop, watch, invest, read, eat, protest, empathize, and perform have all been dramatically, radically overhauled. We do things more quickly, we tend to do more things in the first place because we think we can squeeze more into our digital days, and we have quickly internalized new rhythms of convenience and gratification of pretty much our every whim as normal.

Just as we are getting used to this acceleration and compression of so many aspects of our lives, and frankly learning how to hold ourselves together under the new pressures they bring as well as navigate these new pleasures, we are also beginning to understand that not everything does change so quickly. In fact, there are some aspects of our lives that change very slowly indeed, and for good reason, even if we chafe with frustration at their slower rhythms and routines.

Stewart Brand, an innovative thinker in this new digital age, came up with a clever way to explain this odd, but terribly important feature of the way our lives, and the big systems of commerce, community, and care on which we rely, actually change. He called this framework the 'pace layers of change' (see Fig. 3.4). And like all good ideas, it is both simple and complex.

In Brand's concept, there are six 'pace layers' whose different speeds and rhythms of accommodating change are what makes the overall change process as exciting and unpredictable as it invariably is frustrating and confusing. Change is a function, he argued, not so much of how each layer changes, but how the pace of change in each layer impacts, and is impacted by, the pace of change of the other layers.

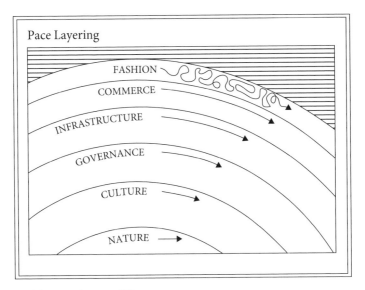

Fig. 3.4 The Pace Layers of Change

Reproduced from Davies SC, Annual Report of the Chief Medical Officer, 2018. Health 2040 – Better Health Within Reach, Copyright (2018), Department of Health and Social Care. Reproduced under the Open Government Licence v3.0.

So, what do each of those layers mean and what goes on in each of them? The explanation below is quoted from a study whose purpose was to understand how the pace layers model might apply in the work of education [9]:

- The fastest layer, **fashion-art,** moves in minutes and months. It is irreverent, engaging, and self-preoccupied. At this layer, a society's culture is set free to experiment, albeit sometimes irresponsibly, learning through creativity and failure.
- The barrage of ideas and propositions generated from the fashion layer gets sorted out at the **commerce layer.** Whether at age-old bazaars or modern-day stock markets and digital crossroads such as Etsy and eBay, commerce brings people together to make sense of new ideas that capture our attention. Commerce tames and harnesses the creative energy of fashion so that society can benefit from it.
- In turn, **infrastructure** changes more slowly than commerce. It is high-cost, high-yield, and delivers delayed payback to society. It provides

foundations and platforms for society to operate—among them transportation, communication, energy, and education. It is refreshed and modernised through the innovations from upper layers while being protected and validated through governance and culture.

- Moving down a layer, the job of **governance** is to serve the larger, slower good for society. It provides stability. It preserves what we hold to be necessary and true. As Brand points out, social and political revolutions want quick change, demanding that governance moves faster than it is capable of, frustrating society. The constraints of governance force reflection and pause, which can be paralysing or empowering.

- Even slower to change, **culture** is the essential work of people as they gather to make sense of and integrate the many facets of life together on earth. It includes religion, language, and the enduring behaviours and social norms that help to provide constancy across centuries.

- The slowest-changing layer is **nature**, with the earth and the human body changing slowly over millennia. Nature's power is immense when unleashed, whether as the processing capacity of the human brain or as the magnitude of earthquakes and hurricanes.

Thinking how this model of the simple but complex way in which human systems change might apply to health and social care is a useful tool for underscoring why health matters so much in the first place.

Starting with nature, the slowest layer, we understand that our health and the patterns of disease and our responses to them are a function of the interaction between the natural environment—air, water, land, forests, and plants—and our human bodies as they have evolved over thousands of years. If COVID-19 has taught us anything, it has taught us, rather brutally, what happens when our lives collide with these slow moving and intense changes in the interaction between human lives and nature.

Culture changes faster than nature because it is the outcome of human interactions and decisions, about patterns of behaviour and thought that can be influenced, adapted, and changed. But it is not rapid or easy. In fact, in many ways, we want culture to be steady and relatively unchanging because it is often the source of habits, insights, and rules that can keep us safe and keep us healthy. Or, of course, exactly the opposite.

In health and social care, culture is the way doctors and medical professionals behave based on their beliefs and attitudes and the way they are taught and trained (which is a hugely important transmitter of culture in itself). It is also the way that business, universities, and commercial research work to discover, manufacture, and distribute drugs and medicines. And it is also the habits and beliefs of people and communities, religious, superstitious, or just the accumulated ways of thinking and behaving that hold whole societies together.

These deeply ingrained habits and patterns do not change just because you want them to. You cannot direct or command culture change. But you can persuade and convince and encourage. It takes time.

Governance is not the same as government, but it is part of the same process by which human societies and, more recently, nations and cities decide how they will take decisions, allocate power and influence, and accord prestige and respect, or opprobrium and disregard. In health and social care, governance is crucial because it is how resources are allocated and how big decisions about the purpose and outcome of the work we do in those sectors are made. It is about how we propose to hold to account those who take decisions and invest limited resources.

Governance can move more swiftly, especially when it has to, for example in the face of a pandemic or, less dramatically but often with similarly dire consequences, when there are natural emergencies like bushfires and floods.

In many situations, people can vote and make changes to the structures, processes, and people of governance methods. It might sometimes feel very slow and extremely frustrating attempting to get change through our structures of governance, but it can be done. And it can be done a lot quicker than trying to change human nature or the rhythms of the natural world.

Infrastructure in health is more obvious and easier again to change and adapt to our priorities. This is the layer in our world from which decisions to design and build hospitals emerge; technology is invented, tested, and diffused; drugs are manufactured and distributed; and complex webs of physical, digital, and human communication built and maintained. It is about our workforces and the infrastructure of rules and regulations within which we ask them to work.

Of course, and for the most part, infrastructure decisions are long term and take a while to materialize. Building a hospital, or the Internet, or developing a workforce of thousands are not the work of a few weeks or months, although it is remarkable what can be done in a hurry when speed matters.

But infrastructure decisions are more malleable and susceptible to human intervention and shifting needs and attitudes than culture or governance.

As this brief sketch of the way the pace layers model applies to health shows, one of the features of the framework is that the nearer you get to the top layers, the faster change happens and the more easily our choices and preferences can be rapidly translated from idea to decision and action.

Speed and volatility are characteristics of both of the top layers in the model. At the very top is fashion or art, which is essentially the layer of innovation and play. Here, almost anything can be done at any speed and, especially in a more digital and distributed world, to suit the rapidly shifting tastes of people and communities. This is the world of Fitbits, mobile phones, new ideas about well-being and care, the fitness movement, and diets. By comparison with governance or culture, this is a layer that changes at lightning speed and at the drop of a whim or a passing idea.

Commerce is the layer that has evolved to bring inventions, products, and services to market and to connect fashion and art with people who want to enjoy their beauty, value, or usefulness. This is how people get to buy their Fitbit and link it to social media apps to monitor and compare their performance. It is the layer that holds the work of GPs and other health businesses, of private hospitals, and care homes for the aged. It is the world of pharmaceutical companies and medical equipment manufacturers. It is the layer that buys and sells both the parade of fashion and art or, sometimes, the more enduring assets and capabilities of health and social care infrastructure.

What lesson can we draw from this framework in the context of our central concern to understand better the links between health, society, and the economy?

If health is the arena within which human flourishing and even happiness are forged and sustained, we need to learn how to navigate the complex choreography of these intersecting layers of change as we seek to make changes that will improve access to quality health and social care. We must understand how each layer needs and feeds the others, and how their rhythms and routines ultimately determine how far and how fast we can move to get the changes we need and the results we want —the chance for all to live healthy lives.

We have to choose what we need from our future healthcare system

The NHS was born out of the necessity to rebuild Britain after World War 2, but its current model is no longer fit for our changing world. The COVID-19 pandemic has highlighted just how vital a service that keeps us alive is to society, but what is needed to treat acute, life-threatening illnesses, from location to personnel to equipment, is very different from what is needed to manage long-term conditions to keep us living well for longer.

We need a new framework that incorporates both these aspects of our health. Futures thinking captures several approaches—forecasting, scenario, and impact analysis—to help us think about what that framework should be. It helps us to leverage potential opportunities and also to identify and reduce the risk of challenges.

As healthcare systems around the world rebuild post-COVID-19, this surely has to be the opportunity to not only rebuild resilience into the illness services, but also to take a broader look at everything that affects our health. Only by valuing, understanding, and fully incorporating all aspects of our health, our total health, will we be able to create a healthcare system and wider environment that makes it easy to be healthy, and to live well for longer. In the next three chapters, we examine the drivers and multiple factors that influence and contribute to our health, or lack of health, to better understand the intricacies involved in developing a more equitable health and care system.

References

1. YouGov. The Local vs the national: the NHS comes into conflict with Brexit in terms of voters' priorities. June 2017: https://yougov.co.uk/topics/politics/articles-reports/2017/06/07/local-vs-national-nhs-comes-conflict-brexit-terms-
2. The King's Fund. British social attitudes survey 2018. March 2019: https://www.kingsfund.org.uk/publications/public-satisfaction-nhs-social-care-2018
3. IPSOS Mori. NHS at 70—Public attitudes to the health and care system. May 2018: https://www.ipsos.com/ipsos-mori/en-uk/nhs-70-public-attitudes-health-and-care-system
4. The Health Foundation. Care homes have seen the biggest increase in deaths since the start of the outbreak. May 2020: https://www.health.org.uk/news-and-comment/charts-and-infographics/deaths-from-any-cause-in-care-homes-have-increased
5. Fertility Fairness. Fertility Fairness Audit. Novemebr 2018. Accessed via: https://fertilitynetworkuk.org/fertility-fairness-audit/
6. Joyce R. Benefits Spending: Five charts on the UK's £100bn bill. March 2019. Accessed via: https://www.bbc.co.uk/news/business-47623277
7. Webster, B. Cleaner air saves around 1,750 lives around country. The Times. April 2020: https://www.thetimes.co.uk/article/cleaner-air-saves-1-750-lives-around-country-pcqtcvc6k?shareToken=01e88564f46480f32d3811c701d e7c62

8. Dahlgren G, Whitehead M. *European strategies for tackling social inequities in health: Levelling up part 2*. World Health Organization Regional Office for Europe. 2006: https://www.euro.who.int/__data/assets/pdf_file/0018/103824/E89384.pdf

9. Saveri A. Reframing education for the long now. *Medium*. December 2017: https://medium.com/the-long-now-foundation/reframing-education-for-the-long-now-3b3672d4f724

4

The social drivers of health

The social determinants of health are the conditions in which
people are born, grow, live, work and age. These circumstances are
shaped by the distribution of money, power and resources at global,
national and local levels. The social determinants of health are
mostly responsible for health inequities – the unfair and avoidable
differences in health status seen within and between countries.

World Health Organization. Social Determinants of Health.
Accessed via: https://www.who.int/social_determinants/
sdh_definition/en/

The conditions into which we are born set off a chain of complex, interlinked responses to the world around us that combine to influence our entire life course. These social determinants, as indicated by the WHO definition, include housing conditions, schooling, the education levels of our parents, employment opportunities, and availability of healthcare. They are traditionally thought of as difficult to change or reset, indeed some are structural, but we think of them as drivers, things that can be changed if the will is there.

We have known that these social drivers contribute to health inequalities for decades. The evidence is well documented and recognizably socially patterned, being worse the more deprived you are. The starkest reminder is the so-called 'health gap'. The most deprived groups experience the poorest health outcomes and these are considerably worse than their more affluent peers. The more deprived you are, the fewer years you can expect to live, and even fewer of those can be expected to be in good health; in England, women in the poorest decile live eight years fewer than those in the most affluent decile, and for men the figure is nine years.

This situation has worsened over the past few decades. The gap between the haves and have nots, between the poorest and richest, has increased, despite improvements to the population average. This has coincided with a widening gap in health outcomes; the more deprived you are, the more likely you are to suffer from obesity, diabetes, heart disease, cancer, or depression. Most

Whose Health Is It, Anyway? Dame Sally C. Davies and Jonathan Pearson-Stuttard, Oxford University Press (2021).
© Oxford University Press. DOI: 10.1093/oso/9780198863458.003.0004

strikingly in England today, at every age and for every disease, the more deprived you are, the higher the chance of dying from that disease at any point
in life.

But we have yet to translate this knowledge into meaningful, feasible action across the board to change things for the better, because too often health
has been viewed in a silo, separate from the rest of the dynamic, changing environment that surrounds it. There is a clear economic case for communities
and nations to address the inherent unfairness in the social drivers of health.
Reducing the health gap between the richest and poorest would go some way
to achieving a more prosperous future for us all; a healthier population is a
more prosperous nation.

In this chapter, we flag some of the traditional social drivers and discuss
several that are emerging. They all present a key challenge; how do we make
meaningful changes to address these social drivers in our ever-changing,
fast-paced world?

The social drivers of health are complex and intertwined

It is impossible to discuss the social drivers of health independently. Housing
affects health affects learning and child development affects later employment possibilities; employment of parents affects housing affects food security affects health, and so on.

The development and learning of a child has important impacts on health
during childhood and therefore throughout the rest of life. The reverse is also
true; health affects learning, and together, they exert a substantial influence
on an individual's future work opportunities and prosperity.

At its simplest, ill health impacts upon an infant's social development.
Even something as basic as a lack of dietary iron, which gives rise to anaemia,
reduces brain development and learning capacity, and subsequently IQ.
A useful indicator is the state of being school-ready; when a child is physically, socially, and intellectually ready to engage and benefit from the learning
environment. This measure has improved in England over recent decades,
though sadly significant inequalities still exist.

Free school meals are a means-tested benefit for children from low-
income backgrounds, hence often used as a proxy for socio-economic status.
In 2016, around one-third of all children aged four years old in England were

not school-ready, with this being some 50% higher (45.6%) in those eligible for free school meals compared with those who were not (28.3%).

This disadvantage continues throughout life; poorer health is found alongside lower levels of education and poorer employment opportunities. Specifically, those with lower levels of education are more likely to be obese, to suffer from long-term diseases, and live in poor health, which in turn affects their ability to fully engage in the workforce and have a meaningful career compared with their more-educated peers: 34% of those with low overall levels of education have one or more long-standing illnesses compared with just 22% of those with high levels of education [1].

Social drivers are interrelated; children who grow up in non-working households, for example, are twice as likely to fail exams throughout their education compared to those growing up in working households. And now that education and learning are no longer confined to childhood and young adulthood, this impacts on an individual's ability to upskill or re-train in later life, when their job changes or disappears as we progress through the fourth industrial revolution.

The likelihood of living in good health increases step-wise as income rises. Perhaps not surprisingly, the links with health go much further than the individual worker, affecting the health of their children and future generations, too. Income, and ability to pay, is very obviously closely linked to housing conditions, which are in turn associated with several health problems, including asthma and other respiratory problems, and mental ill health, such as depression and anxiety.

A safe, settled home is the cornerstone in which individuals and families build a better quality of life, access services they need and gain greater independence.
Jake Eliot, formerly of the National Housing Federation.

As the world we live in has changed, so too has the relationship between housing and our health, evolving to include much more than simply the physical condition of our immediate home. Housing is increasingly precarious, with whole families unsure how long it may be until they find a permanent home or how far that might be from their roots. This can lead to several wider health issues. Factors such as absenteeism of children from school; disrupted development due to moving schools regularly; difficulty for a family or individual to put down roots, form relationships, and integrate into the local community; and difficulties finding stable employment are all relevant.

Housing affects our mental, social, and physical health. Children who live in crowded homes are more likely to have mental ill health and do less well at school. Today more than 8.4 million people in England live in insecure, unaffordable, or unsuitable homes. Many elderly people are living in homes that are too big and hard for them to maintain, whilst millions of younger families face the opposite problem. The housing market in countries such as the UK currently fails to incentivize older people to downsize because moving home often incurs large additional costs (such as stamp duty, moving costs, refurbishments), and also because alternative housing options are unattractive.

At the extreme is homelessness, which has dire implications for health. In the UK the average age of death in the homeless population is 45 years for men and 43 years for women, some 31 and 38 years lower than for the rest of the UK population. Drug overdoses account for 40% of deaths among homeless people—a statistic which is on the rise in both the homeless population and the wider population. The COVID-19 pandemic led to the UK Government saying it was 'redoubling its efforts' to make sure everyone was 'inside and safe' [2]—an important move to protect the vulnerable from the virus, but unless the drivers of homelessness are addressed as we re-build from the pandemic, the benefits will be short lived.

A great challenge for societies is not only to provide homes for growing populations, but for those homes to be appropriate for the life stage of each individual and family. In the UK today, one in five homes do not meet the standard of a 'decent home', for example. As many as 25 million homes in the UK are in need of insulation [3], whilst homes in England are among the smallest in Europe in terms of floor space. Individuals and families with the lowest incomes have suffered the highest rates of overcrowding for centuries, but the COVID-19 pandemic exposed this once again. Overcrowding, and co-habiting with elderly relatives and those with chronic conditions, made it more likely that someone would catch the virus and made lockdown itself more difficult [4].

Poor housing conditions are linked to fewer opportunities for recreation outside. Having safe and regular access to green spaces for physical activity has positive links with both physical and mental health; this was amplified during the pandemic when the instruction to 'stay at home' was made much tougher for the one in eight in England without a garden, a rate that is higher still in poorer urban areas [5]. Unsurprisingly, this too is socially patterned, with poorer areas (including schools in the poorest communities) having less green space and fewer playing areas. In addition, people feel less safe in these more deprived areas and so available spaces are used less.

As our health and the world around us changes, the nature of how these social drivers affect us has shifted too. Previously, being in work was a strong predictor of economic prosperity and, along with education, the foundation for social mobility. The data shows consistently that those who are out of work long-term live shorter lives and have longer periods living with physical and mental ill health. This compounds the dependency of our work and prosperity upon our health today and in the future.

But being in work is no longer enough. Shockingly in the UK today, one in two who live in relative poverty, defined as households having less than 60% of the median income, are in working households. The type of work matters, the security of the work matters, and of course the setting of the work matters. Zero hours contracts, for example, may be good for some, for instance giving flexibility to work when you would like to, and to have more than one job, but for most, the trade-off is the reduced job security, which in turn brings increased stress and anxiety.

Social networks

A significant part of an individual's health is embedded in their network. . . One person's obesity can influence numerous others to whom he or she is connected both directly and indirectly.

Professor James Fowler, UC San Diego

Social networks have always influenced health. COVID-19 reminded us all too starkly how infectious diseases pass from one person to another, clustering in households, friendship or work groups, and communities. But we are now identifying new issues related to our social networks, and alarmingly, their influence on health is often not recognized until problems arise.

Obesity is not contagious—you do not catch it—but innovative research on a long-term data set suggests that obesity can and does spread within a social network. We know that your genes affect your risk of becoming obese, as do your parents' diet and lifestyle before, during, and after pregnancy [6]. The environment in which you live also increases the likelihood of being obese. We are learning that when a person gains weight, it increases the chance of their friends, siblings, and partners gaining weight too.

The research found that the closer the relationship, the higher the chance of gaining weight, with a 57% chance of becoming obese when a close friend is obese. The authors of the research concluded that, when a member of a social group becomes obese, this is likely to change the perceptions within that group about what is a normal body size and weight. Members of the group then adjust their expectations, which results in subtle changes in behaviour and consequently increases the likelihood of those in the group gaining weight [7].

This insight emphasizes the importance of re-shaping our whole environment to normalize healthy, rather than unhealthy, behaviours, which, as the interlinked social drivers above indicate, involves commerce, governments, and citizens.

Social media

Social media is training us to compare our lives instead of appreciating everything we are. No wonder why everyone is depressed.

Bill Murray

Social media and their platforms are innovations that have changed the way we live, interact, and socialize—with profound direct and indirect challenges and opportunities for our health. Social media has followed the World Wide Web as a disruptive force on our lives like no other over the past decade. It has taken social networks online, facilitating new links, networks, and echo chambers. We regularly hear stories about the potential harm that social media and the connected world can bring to our health, but often overlook the potential for benefits.

We in the health world have perhaps been too slow to pick up on this, but is it possible that social media companies ought to have recognized their societal responsibility and considered such issues from the outset? It is not surprising that our understanding of the health effects of social media and the connected world are in their infancy given that it is a relatively new phenomenon. But there is now increasing focus and interest from the public (including parents) and policymakers because social media can be a platform for disseminating harmful information. For instance, anti-vaccination activists (anti-vaxxers) have been active on social media and have found it all too easy to spread misinformation, increasing public distrust of medical authorities and contributing to declining rates of childhood vaccinations.

The role that social media and the connected world has in the mental health of children and young people is particularly important. Several concerns have been raised, including the increased ease of access to a range of unsuitable content that promotes unhealthy diets or body images, opportunistic marketing of unhealthy products, cyber bullying, which can be more relentless than in-person yet less visible to parents or teachers, and potential effects on social development, sleep patterns, and physical activity.

Stories about the links between screen-based activities, including social media, and mental ill health have been increasing in recent years, which has led to increased interest from policymakers and social media companies. The UK Chief Medical Officer published a map of reviews and commentary in 2019 which found that those who engage in social media and screen-based activities more often and for longer periods have a higher chance of mental ill health conditions such as depression and anxiety [8]. Whether these activities cause the health conditions, contribute towards them, or that these platforms are simply more appealing to those with existing conditions is less clear.

Focus groups have identified some of the leading issues for children and young people using social media. They are concerned about: poor self-esteem from comparing themselves against a 'perfect' world captured in social media posts; fear of missing out, or FOMO; and seeking validation for behaviours through achieving a number of likes. This has, in some instances, led to many leaving platforms entirely. A 2018 survey of more than 1,000 people found that over a third of generation Z (born between the mid-1990s and 2010) were quitting social media for good, with 41% saying that social media platforms made them feel anxious, sad, or depressed. Users voting with their feet have increasing influence over the sector, even if they do not realize it.

In many ways it is less important whether screen-based activities and social media directly cause mental health conditions or cluster with harmful behaviours, and more important that we make the online environment as safe and supportive a place as possible for all children and young people to engage and develop.

This raises three key issues for tackling emerging social drivers. First, this is an example where innovations in the world around us outpace regulations that are designed to protect citizens. This can leave people vulnerable, often children in this instance.

Second, the artificially low tax rates that many social media or internet-based companies pay are often at odds with their societal impact. Health is a global good, therefore governments around the world need to work together to realign the incentives around the quality and safety of the experience for the user, and social contributions from the companies themselves. We should not focus simply on screen time; the proposed 'tech tax' is a promising first step.

Third, the value of the data currently held by social media companies is generally poorly understood by the public who sign up and give their data away. Data should not be hoarded because it has great potential to be used to improve the lives and public services of nations. We must re-balance the contract between the data-owning companies and society in order to deliver a data dividend back to both the users and their communities, whilst at the same time recognizing that data about users are crucial to the revenues and success of many internet-based companies.

Social media for good

> *Aisha is studying for her exams but despite her hard work she is finding the pressure of revising difficult. She worries about letting her family and teachers down. And beginning to show symptoms of anxiety which is also affecting her sleep. Her tutor has recommended an app called 'Stress' which is designed to help students address anxiety around exam time. This is a conversational agent or 'chat bot' that offers cognitive behavioural therapy by identifying when users are engaging in negative self-talk and helping them re-frame their thinking in a healthy way. Beth, the chatbot, has engaged on demand with Aisha at all times of the day and while she is still worried about her exams. Aisha is learning to identify unhelpful negative thought patterns and is feeling more positive about the future.*
>
> Adapted from Harriet Boulding et al from Chapter 14, Annual Report of the Chief Medical Officer, 2018. Health 2040 – Better Health within Reach

Social media and the connected world can, of course, be a force for good. It can increase social contact, reduce social isolation, and enable access to advice, educational tools, and vast sources of information. These positive aspects are often under-reported and definitely insufficiently explored or leveraged.

Research has found that routine social media use, when it is used as part of the daily routine and engaged with positively, has positive effects upon social well-being, mental health, and self-reported health [9]. This benefit increased the more educated the user was, consistent with the social patterning in traditional social drivers. Specifically, those who were more educated were able to self-regulate their behaviour to ensure healthy use of social media. Safe and productive engagement with social media should be a routine part of a child's education today.

During COVID-19, video-conferencing platforms allowed friends and families to be socially connected, even if physically distanced. Physical trainer Joe Wicks held free, daily 30-minute physical education lessons for children on his YouTube channel which needed no outdoor space or equipment, which helped children to stay fit, healthy, and have fun during lockdown.

We have scratched the surface of the potential good of social media, but when rebuilding society post-COVID-19, it provides the platform to do much more. For instance, instead of being designed to keep individuals online for as long as possible, social media networks could be used to combat social isolation and loneliness. We already have apps for dating, the same concept can be directed more towards simpler socializing, telling users which fellow users are close by or online and also keen or able to meet virtually for a coffee, as has become common place during the pandemic, or in person for a walk.

In young people, online gaming has actually been found to help those with conditions such as ADHD, PTSD, and depression. Through engaging during gaming sessions, therapists have been able to discuss and explore reactions to in-game scenarios with 10-12 year-olds more effectively than traditional approaches.

The potential good of social media and the connected world for total health, especially our mental and social health, remains untapped yet could transform lives in coming years.

Addiction

Addiction is far more common than we think. Addiction is the psychological and physical condition that means an individual is unable to stop or control a behaviour, which can be taking, using, or doing something, and around one in three of us is affected. Addictions often cluster, and there are many different forms of addiction, all with risks of great personal, family, and societal cost.

Those with addictive tendencies often have issues with multiple substances, and this can have devastating effects for individuals, families, and whole communities. Alcohol and tobacco addiction are two of the most common and well-known addictions, others include social media and work. Constantly checking our smart phones without realizing that we are doing it, or regularly working into the evening, can be to the detriment of our family and social lives.

There are several established approaches to tackling addiction, combining clinical, social, and voluntary organizations. Alcohol addiction, for example, is often managed through peer-support and fostering a sense of community through programmes such as Alcoholics Anonymous. As new addictions emerge, however, different approaches are needed. The World Health Organization recently defined 'gaming disorder' as a mental health condition, which coincided with the opening of gaming addiction clinics in Asia and by the NHS in England.

Two emerging issues in addiction which pose significant but very different challenges to us all in the coming years are opiates and gambling.

The opioid crisis

We think the opioids are a terrible scandal that should never have happened. The mass over-prescription of these drugs has killed a lot of people and perhaps reduced some pain, perhaps not.
                    Angus Deaton, Economics Nobel Laureate

Opioids are very strong painkillers originally derived as morphine from poppies, but now synthesized in laboratories. They are routinely used in healthcare for severe pain for a short period, such as after a road traffic accident, immediately after major surgery, or during childbirth. They are all illegal outside the healthcare context, highly addictive, and not intended for long-term use. Morphine is the original prescription drug and has very similar characteristics to the synthesized drug heroin, whilst fentanyl, a newer synthesized version, is 50 to 100 times stronger than either.

Today, more people than ever are living with chronic pain. As many as one in four or even one in three Americans are thought to suffer. Chronic pain has many causes, from toothache and musculoskeletal backache to pain caused by some cancers. It can be a very difficult condition to deal with and often there is no cure. The physician hopes to minimize the effects of pain on a person's life so that they can cope day to day, but pain can be crippling.

As more people live with chronic pain in the USA, both legal prescriptions and illegal opioid drug use have increased. This has led to a dramatic increase in opioid-related deaths. In 2000, 10,000 American deaths were attributed to opioid use; this increased sevenfold to 70,000 by 2018, with the majority of these deaths being middle-aged men, despite higher use in women (see Fig. 4.1).

Opiate addiction, suicide, and alcoholic liver disease are collectively known as 'diseases of despair', and we have seen a dramatic increase in deaths related to these over the past 10 years. This has contributed to life expectancy in the US falling for three years in a row—a phenomenon not seen since World War 2. There is growing concern that these trends are now being mirrored in the UK, albeit not yet at the same levels. The recession that will inevitably follow the COVID-19 pandemic risks fostering the type of economic and social conditions that have been linked to the emergence of the US opioid crisis; without action this will worsen entrenched unfairness.

Gambling

It's like asking a recovering alcoholic to spend all his (or her) time in a pub or brewery.

Joey Barton, former Premier League footballer

Gambling, for the vast majority, is the odd flutter on an annual day out at the races or a bet on your local football team; 46% of British people report that they have gambled in some way during the last four weeks, at an average of £2.57 per week, or £133 per year. The most popular form of gambling in the UK is the National Lottery (20% of British citizens say they have bought lottery tickets in the last four weeks), followed by scratch cards (11%), and sports betting (7%). The gambling industry itself is big, with £14.5 billion annual revenue in the UK in 2018 and 106,000 employees. Sadly though, gambling is problematic for some, and 0.7% of the UK population are problem gamblers. Gambling addiction is estimated cost the UK up to £1.2 billion per year.

Problem gambling is not new; it is devastating for those affected, and they often resort to lying to conceal the extent of the problem from family,

(a)

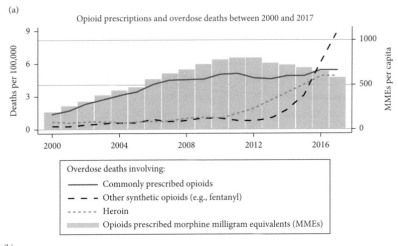

(b)

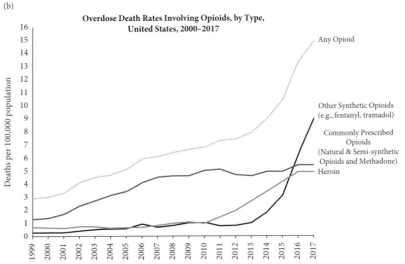

SOURCE: CDC/NCHS, National Vital Statistics System, Mortality. CDC WONDER,
Atlanta, GA: US Department of Health and Human Services, CDC; 2018.
https://wonder.cdc.gov/.

Fig. 4.1 Opioid prescription and related deaths in the USA from 2000 to 2016

Fig. 4.1(a) reproduced from Schnell M, The Opioid Crisis: Tragedy, Treatments and Trade-
offs, Copyright (2019), with permission from Stanford Institute for Economic Policy Research
(SIEPR); Fig. 4.1(b) reproduced from Hedegaard H, Miniño AM, Warner M, Drug Overdose
Deaths in the United States, 1999–2017. NCHS Data Brief, no 329. Copyright (2018), National
Center for Health Statistics.

partners, and friends. The media regularly reports on problem gamblers who steal vast sums of money to fund their addiction, resulting in imprisonment and separation from their children. However, what is new is how the gambling environment has changed dramatically over the past decade, through the exponential growth of internet gambling. With easy access via smartphones, most sports offering in-match betting, and betting markets on almost any aspect of day-to-day life, it has never been easier to place a bet, at any time of day or night, on anything. Online bookmakers also have introductory offers, such as 'bet £5, get £20 free', to make it even easier to get started.

The growing links between gambling advertising and sport share worrying similarities with alcohol. Both see the demographic of sports fans as prime targets to expand their markets; advertising via television during sports events and shirt or stadium sponsors have become commonplace for both industries. When footballer Joey Barton was banned from football for 18 months after being found guilty of betting on football matches (which is prohibited for players), he noted that the Football Association itself had a complicated relationship with the gambling industry. The fact that the Football Association is dependent upon gambling is at odds with its own rules and wider societal responsibility.

> *Buying a loot box is playing a game of chance and it's high time the gambling laws caught up.*
>
> Department for Digital, Culture, Media and Sport House of Commons Select Committee

The rise of online gaming—'skin betting'—is much less familiar, but threatens to be a worrying emerging social driver of children's health. We fear that the mechanisms underpinning loot boxes and skin betting are very similar to those involved in gambling. Skin betting is normalizing gambling behaviour in children and offering a potential gateway into problem gambling later in life.

Loot boxes can be bought using in-game virtual currency that is earned during playing time, or alternatively through purchasing loot boxes online with real currency. Loot boxes contain randomized rewards such as a 'skin' that can change the appearance of an in-game character, or a functional element to enhance a character's performance. These loot boxes are commonplace in online games such as the hugely popular *Fortnite*.

The contents of each loot box is apparently randomly allocated, and the possible prizes, or contents, have a great range of values assigned to them. The rarer skins are worth many times more than those that are more common. Skins from the loot boxes are then used for skin betting, whereby the skins are used as poker chips to gamble online on real-life events. In turn, these skins can be bought or sold online through third parties. A recent report identified several cases of children stealing a parent's credit card to spend thousands of pounds purchasing loot boxes and skins.

This industry has grown rapidly. Nine in ten young people report loot boxes being available on the games that they play, with 40% having paid to open one [10]. Nearly a third of all teenagers in England are aware of skin betting, and 10% of them (around 500,000 young people) report having taken part in skin betting in one form or another. The loot box market is estimated to be worth more than £700 million in the UK, and the global combined market of loot boxes and skin betting is forecast to reach $50 billion by 2022.

This could have devastating and long-term consequences for children and young people. The Netherlands and Belgium have adopted the view that loot boxes violate their gambling laws, and have consequently introduced a number of regulations with the purpose of protecting gamers (predominantly children and young people). In the UK, however, loot boxes and skin betting are yet to be deemed officially as gambling. We believe that governments should protect those who are vulnerable, particularly children. While regulators fail to catch up with the innovations of the online world, our children are left in danger.

Sleep

The decimation of sleep throughout industrialized nations is having a catastrophic impact on our health, our wellness, even the safety and education of our children. It's a silent sleep lost epidemic. It's fast becoming one of the greatest challenges we face in the 21st century.

Professor Matthew Walker, University of California, and author of *Why we sleep*, TED talk Vancouver 2019.

Sleep has not commonly been considered a social driver of health. We usually only hear about its health effects in the more extreme and short-term conditions such as insomnia. It is difficult to study; how many hours of sleep we have is easy to track, but the quality of sleep, and how it affects our health in the longer term, is difficult to tease out. Unlike several other social drivers of health, sleep is often perceived as less easy to change, and lower levels of sleep have conversely historically been associated with perceptions of success, with former UK Prime Minister Margaret Thatcher famously having slept just four hours a night whilst in office.

We are learning that sleep, a state in which we spend a third of our life, appears to have greater influence on our health throughout life than we previously thought. This matters more as we are living longer.

People often assume that sleep deprivation is only relevant for those who suffer with insomnia, living on just two or three hours of sleep a night. A growing body of research suggests, however, that getting less than seven to nine hours of good quality sleep across similar times each night can have serious detrimental effects on our health. Poor sleep is linked with poor health in the immediate and longer term, including lower learning potential, poorer ability to perform day-to-day tasks, and being more forgetful. As far as learning is concerned, sleep is important not only to embed learnings from the day gone by, but also to refresh the brain so it is ready to absorb new learnings the next day. Not enough and poor sleep increases the risk of several serious and common conditions including doubling the risk of heart attack, stroke, dementia, cancer, and premature ageing. And in the medium term, men who sleep just five to six hours a night tend to have the virility of men ten years their senior.

As with so much about COVID-19, the crisis is affecting people very differently depending on their circumstances, and that includes the most fundamental aspects of life, such as sleep.

Professor Bobby Duffy, King's College London.

The best sleep routine is to have similar sleep hours each night so that our bodies can become used to a regular sleep-wake cycle, often called 'sleep hygiene.' Noise and light pollution as well as working patterns all affect sleep. The evidence of the harm related to night shifts, common in factory workers, lorry drivers, and many in the health and care sector, is sufficient for the International Agency for Research on Cancer to classify it as 'probably a carcinogen' [11].

All of the factors that affect sleep, unsurprisingly, are worse in poorer communities. Noise and light pollution are worse in more densely clustered housing, which is more common in deprived communities. The majority of those doing shift-work are lower earners and from poorer communities. More than half of the UK population reported sleep problems during lockdown and it was more common in those suffering financial hardship [12].

Our world is a shared world

The social drivers of health, old and new, are intrinsically linked to the world around us and affected by governments and industry, even when these seem far removed from health. Much of the unfairness in total health is underpinned by the social drivers, and, as total health has become more central to prosperity and happiness, they drive and entrench unfairness from cradle to grave. But we know that there are opportunities for change, and the time is now. Rebuilding total health and society post COVID-19 for a more prosperous future without tackling the social drivers will not work. Improving the total health of the poorest fastest is the only way to level up society after the tragedy of the pandemic.

References

1. Cribb J, Norris Keiller A, Waters T. *Living standards, poverty and inequality in the UK: 2018*. IFS: London. 2018.
2. BBC. All rough sleepers in England 'to be housed'. March 2020: https://www.bbc.co.uk/news/uk-politics-52063939
3. BBC. UK must insulate 25 million homes. February 2017: https://www.bbc.co.uk/news/business-39107973
4. Tinson A. Overcrowding is highest for those with low incomes. COVID-19 chart series. Health Foundation. May 2020: https://www.health.org.uk/news-and-comment/charts-and-infographics/overcrowding-is-highest-for-those-with-low-incomes
5. Office for National Statistics. One in eight British Households has no garden. May 2020: https://www.ons.gov.uk/economy/environmentalaccounts/articles/oneineightbritishhouseholdshasnogarden/2020-05-14
6. Sharp G, Lawlor D. Paternal impact on the life course development of obesity and type 2 diabetes in the offspring. *Diabetologia*. 2019;62(10): 1802–10. doi:10.1007/s00125-019-4919-9
7. Christakis N, Fowler J. The spread of obesity in a large social network over 32 years. *N Engl J Med*. 2007;357(4):370–79. doi:10.1056/NEJMsa066082

8. UK Chief Medical Officers. UK Chief Medical Officers' commentary on screen time and social media map of reviews. Department of Health and Social Care. February 2019.

9. Bekalu M, McCloud R, Viswanath K. Association of Social Media Use With Social Well-Being, Positive Mental Health, and Self-Rated Health: Disentangling Routine Use From Emotional Connection to Use. *Health Education & Behavior*. 2019;46(2_suppl): 69S–80S. https://doi.org/10.1177/1090198119863768

10. The Royal Society for Public Health. Skins in the Game: A high stakes relationship between gambling and young people's health and wellbeing? December 2019.

11. IARC Monographs Vol 124 group. Carcinogenicity of night shift work. *Lancet Oncol*. 04 July 2019.

12. BBC. Coronavirus: How the UK is sleeping under lockdown. June 2020. https://www.bbc.co.uk/news/health-52911395

5

The commercial drivers of health

Efforts to prevent noncommunicable diseases go against the business interests of powerful economic operators.
Dr Margaret Chan, Former Director-General of the
World Health Organization

Companies, especially multinationals, influence our health in a number of ways, ranging from their effect on the physical environment to their influence on government policy and the marketing strategies they use to promote their products in search of profit. The increasing reach and power of multinationals across all industry sectors in recent years has led to an increase in the extent to which they shape our environments and health behaviours, and this relationship is only becoming more intertwined.

The commercial drivers of health are generally defined as factors that influence health which stem from the profit motive [1]. There are many commercial drivers of health, but the connotation is largely negative, with food, alcohol, and tobacco being the leading contributors to ill health and lost years of prosperity.

Our current food system incentivizes volume and unhealthy diets, which, coupled with our sedentary lifestyles, has created what is referred to as an 'obesogenic' environment. Not only has this obesogenic environment led to dramatic increases in rates of obesity, but in turn it has fuelled an unprecedented rise in cases of diabetes, since obesity is a major driver of this disease. These two conditions, obesity and diabetes, are now among the biggest challenges facing health systems and economies around the world.

Alcohol abuse is associated with physical and mental health problems, violence, road traffic accidents, and crime, whilst tobacco is strongly linked to a number of diseases, particularly cancer and liver disease. Hence the commercial imperative to sell these dangerous products puts corporate incentives directly at odds with the well-being of consumers.

Whose Health Is It, Anyway? Dame Sally C. Davies and Jonathan Pearson-Stuttard, Oxford University Press (2021).
© Oxford University Press. DOI: 10.1093/oso/9780198863458.003.0005

However, despite these negative connotations, the food, alcohol, and tobacco industries are highly skilled at making consumers desire their products, and redirecting those skills towards healthier outcomes is complex.

Creating a mutually beneficial relationship between a company's products and the health of its customers requires the right incentives and policies to be put in place when the company is not willing to adopt these independently. These incentives can come from government through legislation, or from consumers voting with their feet and refusing to support companies they view as unethical or promoting unhealthy products or lifestyles.

The COVID-19 pandemic has demonstrated just how vulnerable populations are when obesity and its associated illnesses are rife, and when alcohol abuse and smoking are common. Current data suggest that obese patients who contract the virus have a 30% higher risk of dying, rising to 130% for those who are morbidly obese, whilst those with uncontrolled diabetes have more than double the risk of dying [2]. And the fact that deprived communities are more likely to have higher rates of alcoholism and smoking serves to highlight the dangers of sustaining entrenched unfairness across society, pandemic or no pandemic.

This chapter explores how the food and soft drink, alcohol, and tobacco industries serve as commercial drivers for ill health, and describes examples of legislation aimed at shifting the dial towards better outcomes for all. We also look at the role of individual consumers in shaping our society. Alongside governments and multinationals, 'new power'—the combination of social movements, social media, and purpose—is already re-shaping the world around us, empowering citizens and giving us cause for optimism.

Food, glorious food?

Food is essential to life. One of the great successes of the 20th century was the global effort to tackle food insufficiency, reducing food poverty and hunger around the world. Much work remains to be done to eradicate hunger completely, but the leading food issues facing many countries today are of excess—too much unhealthy food with too many calories, sugar, and salt. When tackling hunger we wanted food production to become faster and cheaper, and for supply chains to make availability a non-issue. But an unintended consequence is that many of these entrenched and incentivized approaches are now driving the epidemic of chronic diseases due to obesity and unhealthy diets. The food system is broken—instead of a platform for health, it is making it harder for individuals and nations to be healthy, costing them their quality of life and prosperity.

The relatively nuanced relationship between food and health is one of the most challenging issues across society today—we need food to survive. Quantity matters, but so does quality and composition, since too much of the wrong stuff is bad for our health. Our understanding of the science continues to evolve too. Nutrition science, studying the links between food, nutrients, and chronic disease, is a relatively new field. Pubmed, the online search engine for Medline, which indexes published scientific articles, shows a more than five-fold increase in the annual number of scientific publications about diet or nutrition since 1980.

The health effects of smoking are relatively straight forward to study, since whether an individual smokes (yes or no), how long for (number of years) and how much (how many cigarettes per day), is clear, but nutrition is more challenging. We do not have to smoke, but we do have to eat. And what we eat matters. One cheeseburger meal can have quite a different nutrient (hence health) profile to another. Once we have eaten the cheeseburger, how it affects us often varies according to our metabolism, genetics, and microbiome—and for all of these, there is still so much that we do not yet know.

Yes, bacon really is killing us.

The Guardian

The media frequently reports that a given food will give you cancer or heart disease. Often the headlines are extremely direct, like the quote from the British *Guardian* newspaper, but this habit of simplifying quite nuanced findings into sound-bites adds to public confusion.

It is true that eating bacon (or other processed meats) each day increases our risk of several diseases, including bowel cancer, by around 20%. That sounds a lot, and is important when advising on dietary guidelines for populations. But when it is put into real numbers, it looks a little different. For every 10,000 people, we would expect 40 to develop bowel cancer. If those 10,000 people ate a rasher of bacon each day, then 40 would rise to 48. Important finding? Yes. Useful to inform consumers and health policy? Yes. Killing us? Not necessarily. As Sir David Spiegelhalter, Winton Professor of the Public Understanding of Risk at the University of Cambridge explains, 'it is important to put statistics like these into perspective'[3].

The obesity epidemic

The role of food in our society has become increasingly prominent in recent years due to the obesity epidemic. The COVID-19 pandemic has brought this issue into even sharper relief, as emerging data show an increased risk of death in those who are obese, and also suggest that two in three adults have put on weight during the lockdown period [4]—our vulnerability to obesity-related conditions looks set to worsen further.

Almost two-thirds of adults in the UK are overweight or obese under current classifications, owing to eating too many calories, and with these calories largely coming from unhealthy, energy-dense food. At the same time, quite shockingly, more than three million people in the UK are at risk of malnutrition [5]. This paradox is also seen in children, where a significant number are both obese and malnourished, meaning they lack the nutrients to grow, develop, and learn well.

Unhealthy diets—high in sugar, salt, and starch, and low in fruits, vegetables, and wholegrains—are linked with a host of adverse health conditions, from heart attacks to cancers, dementia to high blood pressure. Globally, more than one in every five deaths is due to an unhealthy diet, accounting for 11 million deaths in 2017 [6].

We are regularly reminded that obesity and unhealthy diets 'cost' us all, but the World Bank estimate for just how costly unhealthy diets are is truly frightening. They estimate that unhealthy diets cost the global economy just under US$10 trillion today, a figure likely to more than quadruple by 2030 [7]. In the UK alone, costs associated with obesity amounted to around £60 billion in 2018, equating to around 3% of GDP. The opportunity cost of obesity to individuals, employers, and nations is staggering, yet the upward trends have continued largely unchecked until now.

Dietary patterns are generally improving. In the US from 1990-2012, the healthiness of diets improved by around 10% [8]. The US population are eating more whole grains, seafood, and nuts, whilst eating around half a serving of sugary drinks less each day than 20 years ago. A bigger shift has been seen in where we get our calories from. From 1980-2009, the share of our calories consumed from food eaten at home declined by 15-30%, whereas calories consumed in the out-of-home sector rose by around 70% [9].

It is not solely what we are eating that is driving the obesity epidemic, the size of food portions has increased too—packets of crisps and pizzas have both increased in size by more than 50% over the past 30 years and larger waistlines have become the new normal. At the same time, major clothes chains have resized their clothes in response to their expanding customers, creating the impression that actual size has not changed. We all gain weight with age too; the average adult gains around half a kilogram each year, which may seem small but over 20 years that is upwards of 10Kg.

Governments around the world are waking up to the damage that unhealthy diets are doing to populations and economies. The effects of smoking are generally felt as individuals reach middle age, but obesity is becoming more prevalent in younger generations than previously, and long-term conditions such as type 2 diabetes are now being found in children as young as six or seven years of age, a situation that was unheard of only a few years ago. This erects barriers to prosperity and entrenches, and even worsens, the unfairness in life chances for children. Children aged 10-11 years in the most deprived 20% in the UK, for example, have twice the likelihood of being obese as those in the most affluent 20% [10]. Most worrying, this has worsened by around 50% over the past 15 years [11].

Dozens of countries have adopted innovative approaches aiming to redress the unhealthy environment in which their population lives, many by targeting added sugar. Sugar alone is not responsible for the obesity epidemic, but whilst we all know that there is no silver bullet, added sugar is an easy place to start. Most of us consume far too much of it; teenagers in the UK consume around three times the recommended daily amount of sugar, with soft drinks being a major contributor to diabetes, heart disease, and tooth decay due to the extra sugar they contain, above and beyond what is needed to make the drinks in the first place. Dental caries is the top reason for children aged five to nine years to attend the emergency department of hospitals.

Several countries have adopted some form of sugar tax on soft drinks, often using different approaches and with different effects. The French soda tax, introduced in 2012, taxed the manufacturer of any drink containing added sugar or artificial sweeteners 0.0716 euros per litre, irrespective of the amount of sugar the drink contained. This succeeded in nudging consumers to healthier alternatives in the year the tax was introduced, with carbonated drinks sales falling for the first time in eight years. The size of the tax has since been moved to a sliding scale, with higher taxes for drinks with more sugar per 100ml portion.

The city of Philadelphia in the US introduced a 1.5 cents per ounce tax on added-sugar drinks, again taxing according to the size of the drink, not the amount of sugar. Like the French example, this intervention saw reductions in sales of some 40% within the city itself, clearly changing the purchasing behaviour of its citizens [12].

The UK government took a slightly more nuanced approach with its own Soft Drinks Industry Levy (SDIL). Soft drinks with 8 grammes of sugar per 100 millilitres received a 24 pence levy, reducing to 18 pence if the sugar content was 5-8 grammes per 100 millilitres, with no levy below that threshold. While consumers could and did change behaviour, this approach also targeted behaviour change within the drinks industry through incentivizing them to reduce their sugar content and avoid the levy.

The SDIL was announced in 2016 and came into effect in 2018, and had immediate results. Sugar content in more than 50% of soft drinks was lowered before the SDIL was even introduced. Two years later, sugar content in soft drinks had fallen by nearly 30% despite a 7% increase in sales of soft drinks over the same period [13]. Sugar intake down, industry sales up—incentives were aligned and the UK Government was credited with revolutionizing the drinks industry.

Using fiscal levers to incentivize behaviour change in the soft drinks industry has had much more success than the voluntary approach taken to other sugary products. A five-year voluntary pledge in the UK to reduce the sugar content of a range of products, including cereals and chocolate bars, by 20% by 2020 had achieved just a 2.5% reduction by 2017.

Most of the food and beverage industry are waiting for further regulation, such as the SDIL, to incentivize further innovation. However, citizens and governments are now all too aware of our frailties related to the current system, all too harshly highlighted by COVID-19, and want change. In the UK, 55% of the public are in favour of taxes on unhealthy food or drink [14]. Many companies lag behind, but there are some that are already innovating to keep pace with the shifting expectations of consumers.

Nestlé, the largest food and drink company in the world, cut 2.6 billion teaspoons of sugar and 60 billion calories from their products in three years [15]. The sugar content of flavoured San Pellegrino, a leading Nestlé sparkling beverage, has been reduced by 40% in response to the introduction of the SDIL, however it is their non-beverage products that have seen the most interesting developments. In 2016, Nestlé announced that their researchers had managed to create a chocolate bar in which they had altered the structure of sugar through an aeration process involving sugar, milk powder, and water. The resulting sugar dissolved faster in the mouth and allowed a reduction in sugar content in chocolate bars by as much as 40%. Unfortunately, the first chocolate bar they released containing this new sugar was withdrawn from sale after less than two years due to low take-up by consumers [16].

Nestlé are a vast, multi-national company, with the resources to invest for the longer term. For many smaller or family-run businesses, the investment and time-scales required for this level of research and development are pro-hibitive. If food were medicine, surely we would be incentivizing industry to innovate more widely to improve the health on our plates, and reward those that do?

The rise of veganism

If the world went vegan, it could save 8 million human lives by 2050, reduce greenhouse gas emissions by two thirds and lead to healthcare-related savings and avoided climate damages of $1.5 trillion.

The Vegan Society

Veganism has harnessed so-called 'new power'—a social movement using social media united around sustainability—to influence the food and bev-erage market globally. The movement has celebrity members including pop stars Ariana Grande and Miley Cyrus, and #vegan has around 100 million posts on social media platform Instagram.

Veganism has momentum. The number of vegans in the US has increased from 1% to 6% of the population between 2014 and 2017 [17], and UK num-bers quadrupled over a similar period [18]. Waterstones, a UK book store, re-ported sales of books with the word 'vegan' in the title increasing ten-fold in the 18 months leading up to December 2019. 'Veganuary', where people eat vegan for the month of January, had a quarter of a million people sign up in the UK in 2019, compared with just over 4,000 only five years earlier.

There seem to be several related purposes uniting those who attempt to turn vegan. Sustainability and climate change are often cited as the main motivations for becoming vegan, but polling suggests that health (50% of respondents) and weight management are the leading reasons in those inter-ested in cutting down meat consumption, whilst animal welfare is the leading reason in non-meat eaters [19]. The environment is, of course, a big driver too; around one in four cite this as a reason they are eating less meat. 95% of vegans consider themselves healthy eaters [20] and it is not surprising that estimates have suggested that a vegan diet could prevent millions of deaths a year globally. Many, though, urge caution in ensuring vegan diets are not de-ficient in key nutrients such as calcium and vitamin D.

In just a few years, the vegan movement has exerted considerable influence, changing the behaviours of consumers and therefore companies and the market. Sales of meat substitute products grew more than fourfold from 2014 to 2018 [21], with one in six products launched at the end of this period carrying a vegan claim [22]. Not surprisingly, large multinationals are shifting behaviour to keep pace too, with Danone investing US$60 million in diary-free products and the fast-food retailer Burger King launching a plant-based 'Rebel Whopper' in autumn 2019.

Alcohol

We all know that drinking too much alcohol is linked to a host of adverse physical and mental effects, including cancer, violence, and suicide. What is classed as too much alcohol in the UK is more than 14 units of alcohol a week, with 14 units equating to around six pints of average strength beer or ten small glasses of low-strength wine [23]. In 2017, over 2.8 million deaths around the world were due to alcohol, through causes such as liver disease and cancer, and the majority of these deaths occurred in adults aged 50-59 years.

Alcohol is popular. Globally, on average every individual over 15 years of age consumes around 6.5 litres of alcohol per year, the equivalent of roughly 1 bottle of wine per week [24]. This varies a lot by country and culture, however. The Czech Republic tops the league tables, averaging 130 bottles of wine per year [24], with the UK not far behind, averaging just under 100 bottles. Men drink more than women in every country, but this gap has closed significantly in recent years, particularly in the UK.

We know that binge drinking (generally accepted as more than eight units for men and six units for women in one session) is linked with the most harmful effects of alcohol, for both individuals and society. The rates of binge drinking also vary by culture; 30% of UK drinkers report binge drinking, but other countries, such as Germany, although they have higher overall alcohol consumption rates than the UK, have half the number of drinkers reporting binge drinking (15%).

The ill effects of alcohol are felt hardest by the poorest in society. However, there is what has been termed the 'alcohol harm paradox' [25]. Just over 13% of the UK population earning £40,000 or more each year drink alcohol on at least five days each week, compared with around half that proportion (7.3%) in the lowest income group (less than £10,000 per year). But despite the most deprived populations drinking less alcohol than more affluent communities, alcohol-related death rates are five times higher in men and three times higher in women in the most deprived compared to the most affluent quintiles.

Alcohol has societal costs above and beyond the direct effects on our personal health. Consumption is related to increased numbers of road traffic accidents and cases of domestic abuse; in fact around 55% of all crime in the UK is believed to be alcohol-related [24]. Excess alcohol consumption in poorer communities appears to cluster with other unhealthy behaviours, resulting in drinking patterns in these communities that have a disproportionately harmful effect on the individual's and the community's health. Given the reasons often cited for drinking and the wider occurrence of alcohol-related crime, local approaches that recognize these difficult issues are needed.

Low risk, moderate alcohol consumption meanwhile has historically held an important role in social engagements and social health in communities. Moderate consumption is pleasurable for many and pubs have often been the antidote to loneliness and social isolation. One study [26] looked at nearly 3,000 rural communities in England and found a strong relationship between the presence of pubs and social events and activities in a community— stronger than many other community venues such as sports halls.

So unlike tobacco, the message for alcohol is moderation rather than abstinence, which has proved more challenging to tackle well using the 'three As'—affordability, acceptability and availability—since the messages are less clear. For this reason, responses to alcohol-related harms are some way behind approaches to tobacco. A WHO progress update report in 2017 found that nearly two-thirds of countries have increased the scope and intensity of alcohol policies, but much of this centres around a commitment to do something, or increasing awareness, with only a third having turned this rhetoric into action [27].

Increasing the purchase price of alcohol, as with cigarettes, is proven to be one of the most effective ways of reducing alcohol-related harm to society [27]. Several countries, including Scotland in the UK, have adopted Minimum Unit Pricing (MUP), and early evidence suggests MUP to be effective in both tackling excess consumption and also alcohol-related problems. This approach is likely to have the greatest health benefits in the most deprived communities.

We know different types of alcohol are consumed by groups in different patterns, which allows for opportunities to be more nuanced in balancing true health and societal harm with responsible enjoyment in moderation.

The individual and societal harm of alcohol varies by alcohol type (for instance beer, cider, wine, or spirits) and strength, and taxation is likely to encourage behaviour change in individuals who need it most. The Institute for Fiscal Studies showed how a more tailored tax rate for each alcohol type could be applied, taking this into account [28]. They demonstrated that tax rates derived from the combination of the likely effect of changing an individual's behaviour and the societal harm that a particular alcohol type is responsible for could have a much greater effect on heavy compared to light drinkers. Specifically, differential tax rates could lead to the heavy drinkers reducing consumption and switching to less strong types of alcohol (see Fig. 5.1). They estimated that this multi-tiered approach would have a net welfare gain of £350 million, just below the UK Government's estimate of the costs of alcohol-related hospital emergency department visits [28].

As far as acceptability is concerned, public information programmes to educate citizens about alcohol harms have been used by more than 40% of countries, but with mixed results. We know these are likely to be moderately effective at best, and often worsen unfairness in alcohol-related harm.

Meanwhile, the alcohol industry has, like tobacco, taken advantage of the power of advertising to find and grow new markets.

Alcohol brands, and specifically beer brands, began to associate themselves with sport in the hope of reaching its core target audience, namely older males who didn't respond as strongly to traditional advertising. By partnering with teams and athletes, alcohol brands were able to associate themselves with sports and 'share' in the sporting successes and failures therefore making themselves part of the conversation and building loyalty amongst fans . . . .

Conrad Wiacek, head of sponsorship at Sportcal

Where tobacco advertising has been banned, alcohol brands have stepped in to fill the void. As the most popular and most watched sport in the world, it should be no surprise that football is the main advertising target for alcohol brands [29]. Sportcal, a sports market intelligence company, analyzed alcohol brand advertising in sport and found that 49% of all deals globally involved football, way ahead of American football (8.9%) and rugby union (7.5%). Unsurprisingly, they found that 89% of all alcohol sponsorship in sport was by beer companies. Heineken, the brand with the most deals in sports advertising, was found to have 25 active deals in 2018, including one global deal with Formula One worth over $21 million [29].

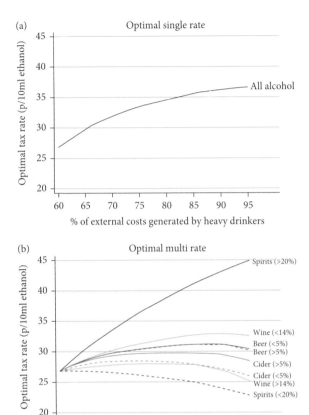

Fig. 5.1 Optimal single vs multi tax rates according to external costs generated by heavy drinkers

Reproduced from Griffith R, O'Connell M, Smith K, Tax design in the alcohol market: IFS Working Paper W17/28, Copyright (2017), with permission from The Institute for Fiscal Studies.

Partnering with reputable or popular bodies to boost public acceptability is commonplace, too. The alcohol industry is perhaps more competitive than tobacco, with a wider range of brands and types of drinks—each often having different target audiences. Companies are expert at harnessing the perception of corporate social responsibility to increase market share or the loyalty of audiences to their brand. One example is the beer brand Bud Light, which provided free beer to all fans when the Cleveland Browns, an American football team, won their first game in over two years.

The generation gap

A new challenge for the alcohol industry is a marked shift in attitudes and behaviour towards alcohol among younger generations. This is causing leading brands to change their approach and products.

> *In 2000, nearly three quarters of teenage Millennials (then aged 13-15) had tried an alcoholic drink at least once – fast forward to 2016 and the figure for 13-15 year olds (Generation Z) is just 36%.*
> Michael Clemence and Hannah Shrimpton, IPSOS MORI Social Research Institute

We are witnessing a shift away from binge drinking in younger generations, and drinking alcohol regularly has declined in each subsequent generation in countries like the UK. Only 6% of Millennials (those born 1981-1996) drink on five or more days a week, around half as many (13%) as Generation X (born 1965-1980) when they were the same age. The numbers abstaining from alcohol altogether are on the rise too; in 2015, 29% of 16-24 year olds in the UK reported never drinking, compared to just over half (18%) of those in 2005 (see Fig. 5.2) [30].

The lower rates of drinking in younger consumers are attributed to several reasons. Focus groups and polling have found shifts in how young people use their leisure time (including social media), greater awareness of alcohol-related harm, and changes in licensing laws as important contributors.

Social media has also provided a platform for finding like-minded individuals to share ideas and support with behaviour change. For instance, 'Hello Sunday Morning', which is a social movement aimed at reducing the stigma around lowering alcohol consumption and encouraging individuals to reassess their relationship with alcohol. Founded in 2009 in Sydney, Australia, it has become the largest online movement for alcohol behaviour change. Founder Chris Raine blogged about his year-long experiment to stop drinking alcohol, signing off each hangover-free blog with 'Hello, Sunday morning!' With over 100,000 members and more than 2.1 million stories shared, the movement aims to support individuals with choosing

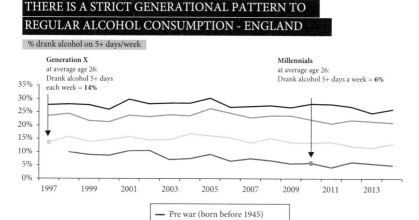

Fig. 5.2 Generational patterns of alcohol consumption in England

Reproduced from Davies SC, Annual Report of the Chief Medical Officer, 2018. Health 2040 – Better Health Within Reach, Copyright (2018), Department of Health and Social Care. Reproduced under the Open Government Licence v3.0. Original source: data from Ipsos MORI, PHE Public Awareness and Opinion Survey, Copyright (2017), Ipsos Public Affairs.

their relationship with alcohol and how it affects their lives. The approach appreciates that preferences and choices are personal, and might be abstinence, taking short-term breaks, or to have a healthy ongoing relationship with alcohol. The programme is mediated through a digital service called Daybreak, which provides anonymous and non-judgemental support to set goals and work with professionals as needed to achieve them. Research published in 2018 indicated that users were benefitting from long-term behaviour change [31].

As with smoking and the move towards e-cigarettes and vaping, these trends have led the alcohol industry to introduce new products to match shifting consumer demand, with some of these products being targeted at non-drinkers. Innovations include low alcohol beers (0.5% ABV), which brewers of craft ales argue retain more flavour than alcohol-free beers, and give the drinker the same pleasurable social experience without the adverse consequences. The sale of low and alcohol-free beers increased by 28% from 2018 to 19 in the UK, with similar trends in other countries such as Germany and Spain [32].

Big tobacco

Smoking or 'big tobacco', is seen by many as the archetypal commercial driver of poor health. It killed around 100 million people in the 20th century [33], more than either of the World Wars or the 1918 Spanish flu pandemic, and continues to be the leading cause of death and disability across the world. Illnesses related to smoking include lung diseases such as emphysema and cancer, heart disease, stroke, dementia, and other cancers. In 2017, smoking led to 7.1 million deaths worldwide.

Smoking costs the UK economy around £13 billion each year and disproportionally affects the poorest in society [34]. It is addictive and harms not only the user but also those in close proximity. These harms extend to the life chances of unborn children. Second-hand smoking causes more deaths than road traffic accidents around the world.

Unless urgent action is taken, we still expect around 1 billion deaths related to tobacco use in the 21st century [35], despite some countries reporting large declines in the number of smokers in recent decades. The big majority of smoking-related deaths in the 21st century will occur in developing countries.

Despite its known harmful effects, smoking is big business. The tobacco market is worth around $1 trillion and supplies around 1 billion customers. In an industry with a seemingly limited lifetime, tobacco companies have harnessed a suite of strategies to maximize their customer base and prevent or delay governmental actions against their products.

Marketing has been crucial to the success of the tobacco industry in its attempts to reach new audiences and pitch smoking as a 'desirable' behaviour. Nearly $10 billion was spent on tobacco marketing in 2017 in the US alone [36]. Sports sponsorship, particularly motor racing, helped encourage smoking among young men, creating apparent synergies between the adventurous nature of motor racing and perceptions of smoking [37]. Such investments reap big and quick rewards; tobacco sponsorship of the cricket series between India and New Zealand in 1996 led to a doubling of the number of Indian children experimenting with tobacco [38].

The grip of tobacco companies on sports sponsorship has been loosened since WHO launched its Tobacco Free Sports campaign in 2002, and advertising tobacco products has been progressively banned at sporting events since then.

As the tobacco market has stalled in high income countries such as the UK due to measures such as banning advertising and smoking in public places, alternatives such as e-cigarettes and vaping have emerged, with many brands of these new products owned by the tobacco companies themselves. Philip Morris, one of the world's largest tobacco firms launched a major UK advertising campaign in 2018 under the slogan, 'Hold my Light'. This campaign encouraged smokers to give up smoking in different ways, including nicotine patches, vaping, and heated tobacco products, all of which are sold by Philip Morris. The campaign circumvented the marketing ban in the UK because it did not advertise smoking itself, but nevertheless was very likely to have similar ends. Leading charity Cancer Research UK accused Philip Morris of 'staggering hypocrisy' [39] pointing out that if the company wanted to cut smoking, it should stop selling cigarettes. Similarly inherent conflicts are found in tobacco-industry funded research, where frequently ambiguous results are cited when calling for a delay in introducing tobacco-related policies.

Although e-cigarettes are marketed as a smoking cessation tool and generally accepted as much safer than smoking, they are not risk-free. The long-term effects of e-cigarette use and heat-not-burn products are unclear. E-cigarettes entered the market in 2003 but it is over the past decade that their use and market share has risen sharply. Tools that help people to stop smoking are of course welcome and needed. However, caution is advised while the evidence catches up, particularly for vulnerable groups such as mothers trying to stop smoking during pregnancy. After all, nicotine is addictive by all methods of delivery. We must remember that it took around 50 years, and millions of lives, to fully understand the harms of tobacco, and decades longer to embed policies to protect citizens; we cannot allow history to repeat itself with these newer nicotine products.

Governments have tackled tobacco-related ill health and deaths through the three fundamental components of any behaviour; affordability, acceptability (and therefore normality), and availability. This comprehensive approach has helped reduce smoking rates dramatically in countries like the UK, from more than 50% of the population smoking in the 1950s to around 15% today.

Governments attack affordability through taxation. Taxes as a share of the price of a packet of cigarettes vary across the world, from 90% in the UK and France to less than 20% in many developing countries. Smoking rates generally correlate negatively with taxation, so that countries with higher taxes on tobacco products tend to have lower smoking rates.

Acceptability is related to cultural factors and behavioural norms, which in turn are influenced by marketing and advertising. Bans on advertising cigarettes have proved effective where introduced.

This approach to reducing acceptability is mirrored by public opinion. When smoking was banned in enclosed public places in England in 2007, the change was supported by 78% of the public. The impact was larger and faster than many anticipated, with 1,200 fewer hospitalized heart attacks in the following 21 months, which in turn positively reinforced the ban.

Availability has been addressed through visibility in the UK. Legislation was introduced in 2012 to ban cigarettes from being displayed openly in supermarkets and later in convenience stores. Subsequent research has indicated that this reduced susceptibility to smoking among adolescents [40].

Despite countries such as the UK having taken steps to reduce the affordability, acceptability, and availability of cigarettes, tobacco remains a threat to global health. We now see tobacco-related unfairness worsening across the world, with developing economies accounting for eight in ten of all smokers worldwide today.

Collective and united action is needed. The 2005 WHO Framework Convention on Tobacco Control represented the first step towards this. Already signed by 168 countries and the first of its kind, the Framework agreed universal standards to limit tobacco use worldwide. This was a major step forward but many of the standards were seen as the bare minimum.

Alongside governmental action, citizens and non-governmental organizations have opportunities to influence attitudes towards smoking and the sustainability of the tobacco industry. Social media has been leveraged for peer support for quitting smoking, particularly through the #QuitforCOVID campaign following awareness of the increased risks from COVID-19 for smokers, which led to more than 300,000 people attempting to stop. Another way public opinion has influenced the industry is in finance and the increasing trend towards ethical and environmental, social, and corporate governance (ESG) investing. Fund managers who adopt ESG investment principles acknowledge that our investments shape our world, and aim to both generate financial returns and benefit, or at least do less harm to, society.

Many large funds have divested from tobacco companies citing concerns around the ethics of tobacco, and particularly strategies to grow markets in emerging economies. These funds include leading players in the pension and investment industry such as Axa and Aviva, and national pension schemes in the Netherlands, Sweden, and Norway. In 2019, the UK's largest pension scheme (the UK Government Nest pension scheme) announced that it would divest all tobacco holdings and not invest in this sector in the future.

Reasons for optimism?

. . . the public are more receptive to interventions than politicians often suppose
The Health Foundation, Nuffield Trust, Kings Fund and the
Institute for Fiscal Studies *The NHS at 70*

Price changes the behaviour of both industry and consumers. This has been demonstrated to be true across all of the leading commercial drivers of health discussed here—tobacco, alcohol, sugary drinks, and food. But as the role of each of these drivers in influencing our health varies, the approach should too. Rather than using blunt tools across the board, data-driven public health approaches would revolutionize the 'polluter pays' strategy in coming decades.

Taxes and regulation are becoming widely accepted in the bid to foster healthy environments, with public opinion playing a big role in government policy. Nine in ten of the British public support sugar and calorie reduction [41], and the popularity of a tax on sugary drinks increased substantially in the months leading up to the UK Government's announcement that it would introduce the Soft Drinks Industry Levy. This approach resulted not only in improved diets, but also in increased sales, showing that fiscal instruments need not be anti-competitive, nor bad for business.

Alongside changes at the macro and governmental level, the citizen's voice has been amplified by the advent of social media. The rise of new power has seen social movements harness social media platforms to unite people with the purpose of controlling their health today and for the future. Younger generations are changing the alcohol industry and markets. Citizens have encouraged the trend for funds to disinvest from corporates marketing harmful products and practices.

These events mark a step change in acknowledging that health and sustainability are global goods and we all have a role to play. Up to now, we have just scratched the surface of this new approach to our total health and there is great untapped potential for continued efforts. We can no longer rely on health bodies and services alone, but we can and must collectively influence the world around us for a more prosperous and fairer future.

References

1. West R, Marteau T. Commentary on Casswell (2013): the commercial determinants of health. Addiction 2013; 108: 686–87

2. OpenSAFELY: factors associated with COVID-19-related hospital death in the linked electronic health records of 17 million adult NHS patients. https://opensafely.org/outputs/2020/05/COVID-risk-factors/

3. Gander K. Processed and read meats are linked to cancer -so how dangerous is a bacon sandwich? *The Independent*. 28 October 2015: https://www.independent.co.uk/life-style/health-and-families/features/processed-and-red-meats-are-linked-to-cancer-so-how-dangerous-is-a-bacon-sandwich-a6711936.html

4. The 1:1 Diet by Cambridge Weight Plan. The UK Lockdown Report. May 2020. Accessed via: https://www.prnewswire.co.uk/news-releases/the-uk-lockdown-diet-report-brits-struggling-as-they-pile-on-the-pounds-reveals-the-1-1-diet-by-cambridge-weight-plan-810594872.html

5. BDA: The Association of UK Dieticians. Malnutrition. Accessed May 2020: https://www.bda.uk.com/news-campaigns/campaigns/malnutrition.html

6. GBD 2017 Diet Collaborators. Health effects of dietary risks in 195 countries, 1990-2017: a systematic analysis for the Global Burden of Disease Study 2017. *The Lancet*. 3rd April 2019: DOI:https://doi.org/10.1016/S0140-6736(19)30041-8

7. Bloom D, Cafiero E, Jané-Lopis E, et al. *The Global Economic Burden of Non-communicable Diseases*. Geneva: World Economic Forum. September 2011: http://www3.weforum.org/docs/WEF_Harvard_HE_GlobalEconomicBurdenNonCommunicableDiseases_2011.pdf 1

8. Rehm C, Peñalvo J, Afshin A, Mozaffarian D. Dietary intake among us adults, 1999-2012. *JAMA*. 2016;315(23):2542–53.

9. Griffiths R, Lluberas R, Luhrmann M. Gluttony in England? Long-term change in Diet. *IFS Briefing Note BN142*. 2013.

10. NHS Digital. National Child Measurement Programme. Child Obesity Profile. March 2020.

11. Davies S. *Time to Solve Childhood Obesity: CMO Special Report*. Department of Health and Social Care. October 2019.

12. Roberto C, Lawman H, LeVasseur M, et al. Association of a Beverage Tax on Sugar-Sweetened and Artificially Sweetened Beverages With Changes in Beverage Prices and Sales at Chain Retailers in a Large Urban Setting. *JAMA*. 2019;321(18):1799–1810. doi:10.1001/jama.2019.4249

13. Bandy L, Scarborough P, Harrington R, et al. Reductions in sugar sales from soft drinks in the UK from 2015 to 2018. *BMC Med*. 2020; **18**, 20 (2020). https://doi.org/10.1186/s12916-019-1477-4

14. YouGov. Do you approve or disapprove of government putting higher taxes on food & drinks that are high in sugar, salt and fat? Plus, obesity, and losing jobs results . July 2019 https://yougov.co.uk/opi/surveys/results/#/survey/e552cbe9-9d6f-11e9-bc29-276664121462

15. Nestlé UK & Ireland cuts 2.6 billion teaspoons of sugar and more than 60 billion calories in just three years. March 2018: https://www.nestle.co.uk/

en-gb/media/pressreleases/nestle-cuts-26-billion-teaspoons-of-sugar-and-more-than-60-billion-calories

16. BBC. Nestlé axes low sugar chocolate due to weak sales. February 2020: https://www.bbc.co.uk/news/business-51439407

17. Forgrieve J. The growing acceptance of Veganism. *Forbes.* November 2018: https://www.forbes.com/sites/janetforgrieve/2018/11/02/picturing-a-kindler-gentler-world-vegan-month/

18. Ipsos Mori surveys, commissioned by The Vegan Society, 2016 and 2019, and The Food & You surveys, organized by the Food Standards Agency (FSA) and the National Centre for Social Science Research (Natcen).

19. BBC. Veganism: Why are vegan diets on the rise? January 2020 https://www.bbc.co.uk/news/business-44488051

20. Moller, R. Is the future of food flexitarian? YouGov. March 2019: https://yougov.co.uk/topics/food/articles-reports/2019/03/26/95-vegans-consider-themselves-healthy-eaters

21. University of Hohenheim. Meat substitutes and lentil pasta: Legume products on the rise in Europe. University of Hohenheim, press release. February 2018.

22. Mintel. #Veganuary: UK overtakes Germany as the world's leader for vegan food launches. January 2019. Accessed via: https://www.mintel.com/press-centre/food-and-drink/veganuary-uk-overtakes-germany-as-worlds-leader-for-vegan-food-launches

23. NHS. Alcohol Units. https://www.nhs.uk/live-well/alcohol-support/calculating-alcohol-units/

24. Ritchie H, Roser M. Alcohol Consumption. OurWorldInData.org. 2018: https://ourworldindata.org/alcohol-consumption

25. Bellis M, Hughes K, Nicholls J, et al. The alcohol harm paradox: using a national survey to explore how alcohol may disproportionately impact health in deprived individuals. *BMC Public Health* **16**, 111 (2016): https://doi.org/10.1186/s12889-016-2766-x

26. Cabras I, Mount M. The importance of pubs in shaping community cohesion and social wellbeing in rural areas of England. 2014. https://www.york.ac.uk/news-and-events/news/2014/research/english-rural-pubs/

27. Jernigan D, Trangenstein P. *Global developments in alcohol policies: Progress in implementation of the WHO global strategy to reduce the harmful use of alcohol since 2010.* World Health Organization Forum on Alcohol, drugs and addictive behaviour. June 2017: https://www.who.int/substance_abuse/activities/fadab/msb_adab_gas_progress_report.pdf?ua=1

28. Griffith R, O'Connell M, Smith K. Tax design in the alcohol market. *Journal of Public Economics.* 2019;172:20–35

29. Christou L. Alcohol brands: The biggest players in sports sponsorship. *Verdict.* 2018. https://www.verdict.co.uk/alcohol-brands-sports-sponsorship/

30. Ng Fat L, Shelton N, Cable N. Investigating the growing trend of non-drinking among young people; analysis of repeated cross-sectional surveys in England 2005–2015. *BMC Public Health.* 2018;18(1090): https://doi.org/10.1186/s12889-018-5995-3

31. Kirkman J, Leo B, Moore J. Alcohol Consumption Reduction Among a Web-Based Supportive Community Using the Hello Sunday Morning Blog Platform: Observational Study [published correction appears in *J Med Internet Res*. 2018 Sept 10;20(9):e11288]. *J Med Internet Res*. 2018;20(5):e196. doi:10.2196/jmir.9605

32. Robinson R. The boom of alcohol free is a sticking trend. *Morning advertiser*. May 2019: https://www.morningadvertiser.co.uk/Article/2019/05/20/How-much-has-the-no-alcohol-category-grown

33. Jha P. Avoidable global cancer deaths and total deaths from smoking. *Nature Reviews Cancer*. 2009;9(9), 655.

34. HM Treasury. *Tobacco Levy: Consultation*. Dec. 2014.

35. Jha P, Peto R. Global effects of smoking, of quitting, and of taxing tobacco. *New England Journal of Medicine*. 2014;370(1), 60–68.

36. Centers for Disease Control and Prevention. Economic trends in Tobacco. Accessed May 2020: https://www.cdc.gov/tobacco/data_statistics/fact_sheets/economics/econ_facts/index.htm

37. Crompton J. Sponsorship of sport by tobacco and alcohol companies: a review of the issues. *J Sport Soc Issues*. 1993;17(3):148–67.

38. Vaidya S, Naik U, Vaidya J. Effect of sports sponsorship by tobacco companies on children's experimentation with tobacco. *BMJ*. 1996Aug17;313(7054):400

39. BBC. 'Philip Morris accused of hypocrisy over anti-smoking ad. 22 October 2018. https://www.bbc.co.uk/news/business-45932048

40. Ford A, MacKintosh A, Moodie C, et al. Impact of a ban on the open display of tobacco products in retail outlets on never smoking youth in the UK: findings from a repeat cross-sectional survey before, during and after implementation. *Tobacco Control*. 2020;29:282–88: https://tobaccocontrol.bmj.com/content/29/3/282

41. IPSOS Public Affairs. *Public Health England: Calorie Reduction Programme Public perception and awareness*. IPSOS Mori. 2018: https://www.ipsos.com/sites/default/files/ct/publication/documents/2019-02/ipsos_mori_phe_calorie_reduction_summary_public_v5.pdf

6

Shared values, shared health, shared prosperity

Public health specialists and policymakers have only recently begun to explore the relationship between commerce and health, what it has been in the past, what it is now, and importantly what it could look like as we re-build society post COVID-19. Alongside the largely familiar commercial drivers of health discussed in Chapter 5, the private sector has several important roles to play in collective health going forward.

The role that work and employers play in our individual, family, and collective health, security, and prosperity has developed over time, and the dependence of companies on the health of their workforce, and their vulnerability to employees' ill health, has changed too. Employers who provide secure employment and safe working conditions for their employees see their prosperity more aligned to the health of the workforce than ever before as chronic diseases (both physical and mental) in working-age people have become an increasing factor in productivity. Employers offering less secure employment in the form of zero-hours contracts, which do not include sick pay and other benefits, clearly see their futures less aligned with their workforce. The flexible model of the zero-hours, gig-economy suits a minority, but for most it is the choice of last resort and can have significant health impacts.

The private sector can contribute to health in its immediate community and nationally through the products it promotes and the causes it supports, especially where corporate social responsibility is more than just a cynical marketing tactic. Sectors that are intimately involved in health, especially the life science industry, have contributed a lot to our longevity in recent decades but can do so much more.

A powerful symbol of the relationship between the nation and health during the lockdown phase of the pandemic was the 'clap for carers'. Every Thursday evening at 8pm for 10 weeks, the nation showed their appreciation for key workers, especially those in the health and care sector, by standing on their doorsteps and clapping and cheering. The phrase 'key workers' came to be recognized as referring not only to those working in the front line of

Whose Health Is It, Anyway? Dame Sally C. Davies and Jonathan Pearson-Stuttard, Oxford University Press (2021).
© Oxford University Press. DOI: 10.1093/oso/9780198863458.003.0006

clinical care, but also to those at all points in the food supply chain, public transport workers, drivers delivering essential goods to those unable to go out, teachers keeping schools open for the most vulnerable children, and many more.

We have choices as a society. Both the decisions we make today and those that we put off until tomorrow will have far-reaching effects on the health of all of us, and may reduce the gap between the most and least deprived, or make it worse. This chapter looks at some of those choices and the impacts they might have.

We need more than occupational health

Occupational health is the promotion and maintenance of the highest degree of physical, mental and social well-being of workers in all occupations by preventing departures from health, controlling risks and the adaptation of work to people, and people to their jobs.

The International Labour Organization and
World Health Organization

Occupational health in the UK has made working life safer over many decades. From the first Factory Inspectors appointed by King William IV in 1833 to the Health and Safety at Work Act in 1974, advances in regulations and the enforcement of structures that promote the health and safety of the workforce have greatly reduced the risk of incurring ill health through work. The general approach, however, has been to minimize the risk of illness and accidents in the workplace, rather than maximize the health of the workforce.

We all know that a healthy workforce is better for employers, because it results in happier employees, lower rates of absenteeism, and higher productivity. Unfortunately, as the average length of time an individual stays in any one job has significantly reduced—we no longer expect to work for the same company for life—many employers do not invest in their employees' health today, using the excuse that they will never reap the rewards in the future. The relationship between work and health has evolved, and the relationship between employee and employer must change too.

There are examples from the past where employers have gone above and beyond the minimum. For instance, the food industry has not always been recognized as simply an importer of ill health. In the 19th century, chocolate was perceived as an ethical alternative to alcohol, and some of the first businesses in the confectionary sector were revolutionary in their approach to the health of their workforce and community. John Cadbury and Joseph Rowntree, who were at the heart of the industrial revolution and boom in economic growth in the UK in the 19th century, established confectionary businesses that remain global brands over 150 years later. They were both members of the Quakers (also known as Friends), a faith group that unites around a set of values rather than beliefs, particularly truth and equality. They saw their businesses as an extension of their family, and understood both the role they had as a large local employer, and the relationship between the health of the local community and prosperity of their companies.

John Cadbury launched his eponymous company in Birmingham in 1824. His sons Richard and George took over in 1861. In 1879, concerned for the health of their employees in the crowded and polluted city, and needing room for expansion, they moved production out of central Birmingham to the nearby countryside. Fourteen years later, George Cadbury started building Bournville, a 'model village' where their own employees and others could enjoy a healthier lifestyle.

At Bournville, the Cadburys developed a reputation for fostering good working, living, and housing conditions for their workforce through mutual respect, relatively high wages, and pioneering schemes such as pensions, joint-work committees, and a staff medical service. Sadly, those societally responsible values have been eroded, and the now global brand Cadburys sells products that contain palm oil, contributing to rainforest deforestation. There was further controversy in 2018, when parent company Mondelez withdrew from the Fairtrade organization, which works to improve working conditions for producers in developing countries [1].

Greggs has baked in responsible capitalism

Financial Times

More recently, the fast food chain Greggs espoused some of the same values as the Cadbury brothers[2]. Greggs started out in 1951 as a bakery, but switched to providing sandwiches and other fast food when competition from supermarkets began to erode its share of the bread and pastries market. A family business with a similar ethos to the early history of Cadburys, Greggs has a charitable foundation supported by 1% of its profits, provides free breakfasts to over 35,000 school children during term time, and has a programme of work experience and training for ex-offenders. Their equitable treatment of employees is reflected in a staff retention rate that is one of the highest in the sector.

Alongside this, in recent years Greggs has begun to change the products it sells. Previously known for fast food at the less healthy end of the spectrum, Greggs began to add healthier options such as gluten-free and vegan products. These have proved to be a big hit with customers, and profit margins have risen by 60% since 2013. Sales in 2019 were up 13.5% on the previous year.

Unfortunately, making headline news demonstrates that the Greggs example is the exception and far from the rule. Nevertheless, some employers are waking up—or perhaps re-awaking—to their role in fostering healthy environments for their workforces, but there is still a long way to go.

Workplace wellness programmes are one example of how employers are trying to address this, but the provision varies greatly. The annual Britain's Healthiest Workplace awards developed by the insurer, Vitality, and produced with the think tank RAND Europe, highlight companies who offer substantive wellness programmes to employees [3]. The awards recognize Britain's Healthiest Workplace, Healthiest New Entrant and Most Improved Workplace. In 2019, the annual survey covered more than 120 companies and nearly 24,000 employees, and gathered data on measures companies had put in place for their employees to improve risk factors for common diseases such as smoking, diet, physical activity and mental health.

The City Mental Health Alliance UK is another example. This organization works across the City of London, one of the world's most important financial centres, to transform workplaces into mentally healthy environments. The Alliance works with member organizations across the City to increase the understanding of mental health and ill health, develop skills and mental health literacy, and embed mental health into policies and procedures [4]. Those in the lowest paid jobs and on zero hours contracts are not so lucky; workplace wellness programmes are rarely, if ever, provided for such employees, which risks worsening existing inequalities.

The productivity of a company is more dependent on the health of their employees than ever before. Job hopping—shorter average duration in each given job—has increased among younger generations, which can contribute to a reduced sense of loyalty and commitment between employer and employee. Perhaps therefore, the lack of mass increases in comprehensive wellness programmes to support employees and families to have good health is not surprising. However, given that secure employment and living wages are much bigger drivers of health than wellness programmes, perhaps we should focus attention elsewhere.

COVID-19—bringing out the best in business?

The total health of each and every community is different, but employers, big and small, help to shape it. The COVID-19 pandemic revealed the extent of the relationship between companies, their employees and society and brought out some of the best in the private sector, alongside, unfortunately, some of the worst [5].

During the first phase of COVID-19, the differences in attitude towards employees were made starkly clear. Timpson, the family owned retail chain which provides shoe repairs and key cutting, were quick to announce that all of its 5,500 employees would be kept on full pay while shops were closed. The UK Government introduced a furlough scheme that paid 80% of wages, up to £2,500 per month, for employees who could not work during lockdown, and thousands of companies that were legitimately furloughing workers mirrored the Timpson example and topped up their pay to the full 100% from their own resources, even when the business was seeing revenues dwindle or even halt. Sadly, there are companies that abused the furlough programme, but the vast majority adhered to the restrictions.

LloydsPharmacy, along with many supermarkets, recruited extra employees during the pandemic, not only to keep up with demand from the increased needs of often home-quarantined individuals, but also because they identified an increasing pool of workers who had seen their jobs end abruptly.

During the pandemic we also saw a host of philanthropic programmes across the country. More than one million children in the UK rely on free school meals; when schools were closed during the lockdown, food poverty and hunger were a real concern for many of these children, large numbers of whom were in households with parents whose income was affected. The Co-operative group, a retail group in the UK, provided a £20 weekly food voucher to each of the 6,000 pupils at Co-op Academy schools across the country who were eligible for free school meals. In June 2020, the Co-op announced that it would continue the scheme during the summer holidays [6].

Several fast-food chains made similar contributions. 'FeedNHS' was an initiative which delivered more than 5,000 meals for free each day to hospitals across London, backed by chains including Wasabi, Abokado, and

Franco Manca. Similarly, other food chains, such as Leon, kept branches near hospitals open and provided a 50% discount to those working in the health sector. Supermarkets got in on the act, too, with Waitrose allowing NHS workers priority at checkouts so that they could get home faster to rest, and Sainsburys having periods of their opening times restricted to key workers only.

Large multinational companies also made donations to the pandemic response; the UK division of HSBC donated £1 million to help vulnerable people affected by COVID-19 and Unilever donated nearly £100 million, including £50 million in kind, in the form of soap, sanitiser, bleach, and food.

Innovating together for total health

Innovations in health are often detached from innovations in other sectors. Too often it appears that healthcare in the UK adopts innovations more slowly than other sectors—automation, digital infrastructure, and AI are just a few examples. The almost unique circumstances of the pandemic, however, seemed to reverse this trend. Dozens of companies wrote to the government with offers of help, adapting their innovations from other sectors to help the NHS in the fight against COVID-19.

One of the big concerns at the beginning of the pandemic was whether hospitals in the UK would have enough ventilators available for every patient who may need one. As part of the Formula 1 Racing Project Pitlane Scheme, the Mercedes-AMG Petronas Formula 1 team worked with anaesthetists at University College Hospital in London to design, make, and deliver 10,000 continuous positive airway pressure (CPAP) devices—a machine that helps patients who need breathing support but who do not require ventilation. Adopting their innovations and applying them to the healthcare setting took fewer than 100 hours for the initial version, and the designs were then made freely available to other manufacturers [7]. Alongside this, the UK regulator, the Medicines and Healthcare products Regulatory Agency (MHRA), acted with similar speed, assessing and approving the devices months quicker than would usually be the case.

Another concern was availability of Personal Protective Equipment (PPE). Burberry, the luxury fashion brand, made and donated more than 100,000 items of PPE to the NHS [8], alongside maintaining pay for employees unable to work during lockdown. Mulberry, another high-end brand, also adapted their production process to produce PPE gowns for healthcare workers.

Major telecoms companies, including BT/EE, Sky, O2, and Virgin Media, also stepped in to help. An essential move to reduce the risk of spreading the coronavirus was to transfer as many medical appointments as possible online, via video or telephone link. But, despite many years of discussions, enabling digital services across the NHS and routinely delivering remote consultations was a long way off. The pandemic changed this almost overnight. The big telecoms providers improved connectivity across care homes and within hospitals, and agreed to provide increased internet data and call services to NHS workers at no extra cost, also upgrading the broadband in NHS workers' homes to make remote consultations possible. Within just a few weeks, some primary care practices reported completing up to 90% of all consultations digitally, where previously around 90% of appointments were face to face [9].

Digital companies also responded to a call from government to help integrate datasets across the health system so that the NHS and government had close to real-time information on key issues. This included what, and how much, PPE was within the system and where the greatest need may be in coming days and weeks. Similarly, tracking live activity across the NHS meant being able to better allocate resources as the epidemic curve was different in each region. Palantir, the US technology company, brought together the many datasets through a logic model that could inform decisions each day, and Amazon provided the cloud support through Amazon Web Services. All of this dramatically helped NHS hospitals respond effectively and ensure that few precious resources, from PPE to ventilators, were wasted.

Anti-microbial resistance is a major market failure

If we fail to act, we are looking at an almost unthinkable scenario where antibiotics no longer work and we are cast back into the dark ages of medicine where treatable infections and injuries will kill once again.

David Cameron, former UK Prime Minister

The coronavirus pandemic has brought the threat of infectious diseases to the front of everyone's minds and antibiotics have played their part; many of the COVID-19 patients who end up on ventilators are treated with antibiotics for proven or presumed ventilator-related pneumonia.

When doctors and scientists are asked to list the top medical advances in the 20th century, the discovery of penicillin and antibiotics is always at or near the top of the list. Indeed, WHO has estimated that antibiotics have given us each on average an extra 20 years of life. Antibiotics and other anti-infectives underpin modern healthcare. In their absence, routine operations like replacement joints and Caesarean sections would be highly risky. Without antibiotics, we would have to rethink as a society not only treatments, transplantation, and renal dialysis but much more, because a simple urine infection or scratch could lead to sepsis and death.

But despite the tremendous impact antibiotics have had on modern medicine and their role in treating patients with COVID-19, they are becoming less effective. Common bugs such as Methicillin-resistant Staphylococcus aureus (MRSA) have developed resistance to many antibiotics, leaving hospitals facing real dangers for their patients. Ultimately, antimicrobial resistance (AMR) threatens almost every aspect of modern medicine, from cancer treatments to caesarean sections, and often the only barrier that protects patients from further infection is good hygiene [10].

This is not a new challenge. Indeed, it was predicted by Alexander Fleming, the discoverer of penicillin, but it is now becoming increasingly urgent. Up to 50,000 lives are lost due to AMR each year in Europe and the US. An independent review of AMR in 2016, led by Lord O'Neill, concluded that by 2050, 10 million lives each year would be at risk, along with a cumulative economic loss of $100 trillion worldwide [11]. The World Bank has forecast that, without action, AMR could cause similar economic damage to that seen in the 2008 financial crisis, costing the world around 3.8% of GDP in the worst case scenario and pushing an extra 28.3 million people into extreme poverty [12]. A recent study in Canada showed that AMR reduced their GDP by C$2 billion in 2018 due to its impact on labour productivity. It also resulted in lengthier hospital stays, longer courses of treatment, and other expenses, which cost the Canadian healthcare system an additional C$1.4 billion. The Canadian government forecasts a $388 billion cumulative loss in GDP due to AMR by 2050 [13].

Why are we in this dire position? It is due to a deadly combination of bacteria developing resistance to existing antibiotics and a lack of research and development into new antibiotics. In fact, no new classes of antibiotics have come into routine clinical use for over 25 years, and this is down to market failure.

Today's society incentivizes the private sector to make a profit, almost irrespective of wider societal impacts. The very purpose of the pharmaceutical industry is to make a profit through selling goods that aim to prevent or treat illness and promote health. Worth an estimated $935 billion in 2017

[14], this sector has made great contributions to our health, from developing medications for HIV that transformed the outlook for infected individuals from an early death to a near-normal life expectancy, to delivering vaccines around the world to prevent conditions such as measles and polio.

But the profit motive also means that the pharmaceutical industry is not incentivized to invest the resource and capacity required to tackle AMR. Profitability for pharmaceutical companies is based on volumes of sales—the more drugs they sell, the more money they make. Antibiotics are relatively inexpensive, and used as sparingly as possible to do the job and no more, whereas drugs taken daily for conditions such as diabetes or high blood pressure are much more profitable. To date, no healthcare system or provider has been prepared to pay the same amount to cure an infection as they would pay for novel anti-cancer treatments, even though antibiotics save lives just like drugs that treat cancer.

Thus the pharmaceutical industry is not encouraged to invest in developing new antibiotics because they might prevent the need for other, more profitable drugs, and many companies have divested from antimicrobial research and development as a result. At the same time, a number of small biotech companies with potentially useful antibiotics have gone bust before bringing their new treatments to market.

There is a clear imperative for governments and the pharmaceutical industry to act. For governments, it would mean saving lives and money. For the companies involved, it may ultimately mean maintaining financial viability, since many of their most lucrative products, including novel cancer treatments, will be rendered useless if AMR continues apace.

There is a glimmer of hope—a global non-profit partnership entitled Combating Antibiotic-Resistant Bacteria Biopharmaceutical Accelerator (CARB-X) was set up in 2016 to accelerate research into AMR and the development of new treatments. With $500 million in initial funding from an array of national and international organizations, including the Bill & Melinda Gates Foundation and the Wellcome Trust, to date, CARB-X has invested over $230 million in 63 projects around the world. Big pharma has yet to adopt any of the programmes initiated by CARB-X.

New power—a second front against AMR

Intensive farming methods around the world result in animals being reared and raised under poor living conditions, including inadequate infection prevention and control. To compensate for this, livestock farmers regularly use antibiotics as prophylactics rather than treatments, and, outside Europe, they are also widely used to promote growth. In the US, 70% of medically important antibiotics are destined for animal agriculture rather than human use [15]. Compensating for the lack of biosecurity and poor animal welfare in this way has led to increasing resistance to bacteria, which can and does spill into the human food chain.

Chain Reaction is a social movement instigated by a group of public interest and non-governmental organizations in the US that is using new power to unite consumers around restricting the use of antibiotics in livestock and poultry. Restaurant chains in the US have huge purchasing power and Chain Reaction assesses the top 25 according to their progress in eliminating the routine use of antibiotics among their suppliers. They aim to encourage both consumers and large restaurant chains to consider provenance and sourcing when they choose the meat they eat and sell. Transparent pressure from consumers is having an effect, with Chain Reaction's annual survey in 2017, its third, finding that 14 of the top 25 fast food chains had started taking steps to limit the use of antibiotics across their supply chains and received what Chain Reaction term 'passing grades'. Among the 11 chains graded F were Dairy Queen and Domino's Pizza. Only two, Chipotle and Panera Bread, were graded A [15].

The air we breathe

The biggest tab the public picks up for fossil fuels has to do with what economists call 'external costs,' like the health effects of air and water pollution.

Jeff Goodell, leading environmental journalist and author

Air pollution is a significant cause of chronic diseases, contributing to nearly five million deaths worldwide in 2017 [16]. It causes ill health from a number of conditions, including heart disease, strokes, asthma, and other chronic lung conditions, yet it is only in recent years that this has been recognized. Exposure to outdoor fine particulate matter, $PM_{2.5}$, is the fifth leading risk factor for death and disability worldwide: 16% of all lung cancer deaths, 25% of all chronic obstructive pulmonary disease deaths, and around 17% of all ischaemic heart disease deaths are attributed to high $PM_{2.5}$.

Unfortunately, higher air pollution is generally a by-product of economic development, itself a positive driver of health. Air pollution in the form of greenhouse gases is also associated with climate change, and countries around the world are looking to mitigate these effects. The UK has enshrined into law the target of bringing all greenhouse gas emissions to net zero by 2050.

Many high-income countries have previously benefited economically from their polluting status, whilst many low and medium-income countries are at the beginning of a similar economic journey, and the latter reasonably raise questions of fairness when it comes to international efforts to reduce emissions. Who has benefitted from past pollution and how quickly should each country be reducing emissions? The 'polluter pays' principle suggests that countries which have already benefitted from the activities that caused the pollution in the first place should bear the largest burden in tackling the consequences.

The effects of air pollution are felt unfairly within countries, too. Those with asthma, for example, and the elderly are more affected by air pollution, as are those living in poorer communities.

Progress has been made in reducing emissions, but as with smoking, it has not been felt equally. During the school run, children in London are five times more exposed to air pollution than any other time of the day, but this varies across schools. In 2001 in the UK, 2.5 million people lived in areas where the yearly average NO_2 limit was exceeded; over half of these people were in the poorest 20% of the population. Fast forward ten years to 2011 and, whilst the number of people exposed to NO_2 above the limit had reduced substantially to 0.6 million, 85% of these people were in the poorest 20%. Improvements at the national level mask the growing unfairness inherent in where we are born, live, and work.

It can never be ethically acceptable that people are killed or seriously injured when moving within the road transport system.
The underlying principle for Vision Zero, the multi-national traffic safety project of Sweden.

Societies are committed to reducing greenhouse gas emissions, but a big opportunity will be missed if efforts are not made to redress many of the accompanying contributions to ill health and unfairness. We can learn lessons for this complex public health issue from Vision Zero, a campaign that began in Sweden in the 1990s to reduce road deaths [17]. Vision Zero accepts that human error is inevitable within any system, so systems must be designed to ensure that such faults do not lead to death or serious injury. It integrates safety into the entire process, from roads to regulation, including engineering, vehicle design, driver training, and lighting.

One of the few positives of the COVID-19 lockdown in Spring 2020 was the dramatic reduction in emissions—scientists estimate this led to 11,000 fewer deaths across Europe than would have been expected otherwise during the two-month period. When working towards net zero, rather than solely focusing on the lowest-hanging fruit or reducing average exposure across nations, we must acknowledge that the highest health impacts of pollution are felt in the most deprived communities, so those communities are where efforts should be focused. This break in business as normal presents a real opportunity to reduce emissions by developing and ensuring safe, attractive, and affordable options for active travel across all populations in the post-COVID world.

Physical activity and active travel

Physical fitness is not only one of the most important keys to a healthy body, it is the basis of dynamic and creative intellectual activity.

John F. Kennedy

Regular physical activity protects us from a host of physical and mental health conditions, giving the greatest benefits if sustained over a lifetime [18]. Despite this, we continue to lead sedentary lifestyles, with nearly one in 40 deaths in England due to not exercising enough. Sedentary lifestyles also have significant effects on ill health during our lifetime, and cost the UK economy around £7.4 billion each year, including £1 billion of costs to the health service. As a key risk factor for diabetes, musculoskeletal problems, and common mental ill health conditions such as depression, not getting enough exercise can have big impacts on an individual's productivity and work potential, in turn affecting the wider economy.

High profile sports are often held up as examples when discussing physical activity, and many across the country enjoy participating in sports during evenings or weekends. The easiest and most sustainable way for most of the population to keep active, however, is through active travel, walking or cycling as part of a daily routine to get to work or attend social occasions.

Despite this, we in England were walking 20% less per week in 2015 than in 2005.

Physical activity rates vary greatly across populations. Generally, activity reduces with age, and more women (25%) are rated inactive compared to men (21%) [19], with two million fewer women active than men despite 75% of women saying they would like to exercise more, according to Sport England's Active People Survey [20]. Fear of judgement, stigma around body composition, and ability were cited as contributing factors. Sport England launched the 'This Girl Can' campaign in 2015 to combat this. It harnessed social media through a video showing women of all ages, body types, and skill levels enjoying different sports, and used the hashtag #thisgirlcan. On the first day the advert was aired, the hashtag trended at number three in the UK. Subsequently, the gap between men and women who exercise regularly had reduced to 1.3 million by 2017 and the campaign is credited with persuading 1.6 million women across the UK to start exercising [21].

Physical inactivity and sedentary behaviour are twice as common in the most deprived 20% of the population (34%) as in the richest (17%) in England (see Fig. 6.1) [22]. This is perhaps unsurprising given that people

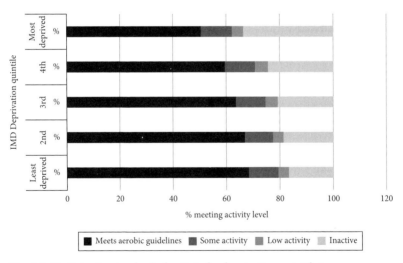

Fig. 6.1 Participation in physical activity by deprivation quintile in England, 2016

Reproduced from Davies SC, Annual Report of the Chief Medical Officer, 2018. Health 2040 – Better Health Within Reach, Copyright (2018), Department of Health and Social Care. Reproduced under the Open Government Licence v3.0. Original source: data from NHS Digital.

living in deprived areas generally have less access to safe green space and/or the means to invest in equipment required for activities such as cycling. Even free activities see inequalities of uptake. Park Run, a free, timed 5 km run that, until the pandemic, took place at hundreds of outdoor venues around the country and around the world every Saturday, has been a great success in increasing physical activity in a non-stigmatizing way. Research has found it to be an attractive proposition to non-runners and a welcoming community [23], although it does appear to struggle with reaching all sectors of the community [24]. This inequality is also seen when cycle lanes are introduced in cities; the costs of buying a bike and equipment are often prohibitive to those on lower incomes, so cycle lanes tend to be filled with so-called MAMILs, middle-class, middle-aged men in lycra.

Behaviours changed dramatically during the pandemic. We have mentioned the huge reduction in car journeys and related emissions, but another development was pop-up cycle lanes. These were put in place to make cycling safer as people were encouraged to use active transport rather than public transport where possible to reduce the virus spread.

As we look to re-build after phase one of the pandemic, this is another opportunity to build in structures and incentives to normalize active travel as part of tackling engrained unfairness and set the groundwork for healthier and more sustainable travel and lifestyle patterns for generations to come.

We're all in this together

Too often the profit motive has not been aligned with societal benefits so that many industries across the commercial world harm our health even when they exist to protect and promote it. Commerce could and should do more. Where governments have attempted to redress this through mechanisms such as polluter pays, the efforts have often been too little or too late to mitigate the harm to society.

A healthy population benefits us all, and we believe that those companies who are realizing this and taking a holistic approach to their role in supporting their employees, communities, and nations will find public and political support is behind them in years to come.

During the first phase of the pandemic, we saw some extraordinary measures from businesses large and small, realizing the societal role they could play to help in this crisis. The direct benefits of this were there for all to see, whether community programmes to feed school children or developing and donating machines to help patients stay alive. This brought the best out of the health sector itself—regulators acted faster than ever before whilst not compromising safety, and much of primary care did truly become digital first.

We can make this the new normal if we choose to. There will be many choices post COVID-19 and this more societal approach from businesses and faster adoption of innovations across healthcare to get the best care to patients without delay will pay off for individuals, businesses, and governments, and should become embedded permanently.

In the next chapter, we examine the more direct challenges for the healthcare system, and the embedded habits and processes that sometimes results in a system that does not function in the best interest of the patient or the individual seeking to remain healthy.

References

1. Nadkarni A. Cadbury's move on ethical trade 'a terrible step back'. *Stuff*. May 2018: https://www.stuff.co.nz/business/103518582/understanding-cadburys-ethical-cocoa-badges
2. Masters B. Greggs has baked in responsible capitalism. *Financial Times*. 20 January 2020. https://www.ft.com/content/6a807f5a-32c2-11ea-a329-0bcf87a328f2.
3. Jack A. Winners of the 2019 Britain's healthiest workplace awards. *Financial Times*. November 2019: https://www.ft.com/content/0ad428d4-0506-11ea-9afa-d9e2401fa7ca
4. City Mental Health Alliance. Accessed May 2020: http://citymha.org.uk/about-us/
5. Partridge J. Which Companies are coming through during the coronavirus crisis? *The Guardian*. March 2020: https://www.theguardian.com/business/2020/mar/29/which-companies-are-coming-through-during-the-coronavirus-crisis
6. Co-op Academies Trust. 16 June 2020: https://www.coopacademies.co.uk/stories/co-op-to-fund-free-school-meals-throughout-summer-holidays/
7. https://www.mercedesamgf1.com/en/news/2020/04/ucl-uclh-f1-project-pitlane-start-delivery-breathing-aids-nhs-hospitals/
8. BBC. Coronavirus: Burberry donates PPE to NHS. April 2020: https://www.bbc.co.uk/news/uk-england-leeds-52415983
9. Ford P. Digital triage changes the game for UK GP practices in the age of COVID-19. *Mobile Health News*. May 2020: https://www.mobihealthnews.com/news/europe/digital-triage-changes-game-uk-gp-practices-age-COVID-19
10. UK Government. Press release: Prime Minister warns of global threat of antibiotic resistance. Department of Health and Social Care and Prime Minister's Office, 10 Downing Street. July 2014: https://www.gov.uk/government/news/prime-minister-warns-of-global-threat-of-antibiotic-resistance

11. O'Neill, J. Tackling Drug-Resistant Infections Globally: Final Report and Recommendations. The Review on Antimicrobial Resistance. Wellcome Trust, HM Government. 2016: https://amr-review.org/sites/default/files/160525_Final%20paper_with%20cover.pdf.

12. Jonas O, Irwin A, Berthe F, Le Gall F, Marquez P. *Drug-Resistant Infections: A Threat to Our Economic Future.* HNP/Agriculture Global Antimicrobial Resistance Initiative. Washington DC: World Bank Group. 2017.

13. Council of Canadian Academies. When Antibiotics Fail. November 2019.

14. Marketresearch.com The Growing Pharmaceuticals Market: Expert Forecast and Analysis May 2018.: https://blog.marketresearch.com/the-growing-pharmaceuticals-market-expert-forecasts-and-analysis

15. Friends of the Earth. Chain Reaction III Report. September 2017: https://foe.org/resources/chain-reaction-iii-report/

16. GBD 2017 Risk Factor Collaborators. Global, regional, and national comparative risk assessment of 84 behavioural, environmental and occupational, and metabolic risks or clusters of risks for 195 countries and territories, 1990–2017: a systematic analysis for the Global Burden of Disease Study 2017. *The Lancet.* November 2018: https://doi.org/10.1016/S0140-6736(18)32225-6

17. Tingvall C, Haworth N. Vision zero: an ethical approach to safety and mobility. Monash University. 1999: https://www.monash.edu/muarc/archive/our-publications/papers/visionzero

18. Public Health England. Guidance: Physical activity: Applying All Our Health. October 2019: https://www.gov.uk/government/publications/physical-activity-applying-all-our-health/physical-activity-applying-all-our-health

19. NHS Digital. (2017). Health Survey for England—2016. NHS Digital.

20. Sport England's This Girl Can, data from Active Lives Adults.

21. Roderick L. New 'This Girl Can' campaign to target 'teens, mums and their grandmothers'. *Marketing Week.* 31 Jan 2017: https://www.marketingweek.com/new-girl-can-campaign/

22. NHS Digital. Health Survey for England—2016. NHS Digital. 2017.

23. Stevinson C, Hickson M. Exploring the public health potential of a mass community participation event. *Journal of Public Health.* June 2014. 36 (2)268–74. https://doi.org/10.1093/pubmed/fdt082

24. Goyder E, Edmonds C, Sabey A, et al. P2 What factors predict participation in a mass community physical activity programme? the case of the five sheffield 'parkruns'. *J Epidemiol Community Health.* 2018;72:A61–A62.

7

Does the healthcare system help or hinder our health?

Whether the healthcare system helps or hinders our health may seem a silly question. After all, the NHS has been crucial in saving the lives of tens of thousands of people during the first wave of the COVID-19 pandemic; without it the death toll would have been many times higher. But is our healthcare system helping us to be and remain healthy in the long term?

Those who have experienced the healthcare system when they have needed it most will testify that 'without it, I would not be here today' and, for those who have had an acute illness or major health scare, this is generally true. The healthcare system treats our illnesses and injuries and gets us back on our feet, whether after a road traffic accident, a broken hip, or appendicitis, so that we can go back to work and enjoy our life. Long-term conditions are a different story, they cannot be dealt with as a single, isolated episode of ill health, and have lasting effects on our ability to live a full life.

Acute illness therefore generally has a far smaller impact on our society and economy than long-term conditions that are not well controlled. Keeping populations living in good health for longer is a very different challenge to treating their (often acute onset) illnesses; it requires different tools, different structures, and different incentives. Treating acute illness and living well with chronic conditions are really quite different. We all need both in different amounts at different times, but our healthcare system currently has neither the right model nor sufficient resilience to do both, despite its remarkable and dedicated workforce.

The unexpected COVID-19 pandemic revealed the precariousness of this situation in the UK. The NHS was not set up, nor was it resilient enough, to cope with normal care and COVID-19 together, partly as a result of years of receiving only just enough funding to keep going. This inevitably left us with the unpalatable choice of turning the entire system over to combatting the pandemic at the cost of other services, such as those treating cancer patients, or trying to tackle COVID-19 alongside business as usual and risk failing at both.

Whose Health Is It, Anyway? Dame Sally C. Davies and Jonathan Pearson-Stuttard, Oxford University Press (2021). © Oxford University Press. DOI: 10.1093/oso/9780198863458.003.0007

Despite the efforts of the health and care workforce, there were more than 60,000 excess deaths in England and Wales in the three months from March to May 2020. Yet the reality is that there are likely to be many more deaths than expected from other physical and mental health conditions over subsequent months and years because the health service pivoted, almost entirely, to focus on the pandemic.

The threat from COVID-19 still remains, and so we must be ready and more resilient for future waves and pandemics. Alongside this, the need for acute care for other conditions does not go away; people continue to have heart attacks, strokes, falls, and road traffic accidents. But when the system is stretched, each winter with flu or by less predictable events such as COVID-19, those with chronic conditions inevitably lose out; more than two million patients with cancer were affected in Spring 2020 due to delays to operations or courses of treatment. Whilst partly due to the capacity and resilience of the NHS, this was also due to genuine practical considerations—immunosuppressed patients, such as those with cancer or transplanted organs, had a greater risk of catching COVID-19 and dying from it if they went to hospital for other treatments because hospitals had the highest circulating levels of the virus at times. If we are to learn to live with the threat of COVID-19 returning or other pandemics hitting in the future, we cannot afford for this to be the case again.

In this chapter we examine the problems inherent in the healthcare system today, and explore what a health system that helps us live well might look like. We examine the incentives and structures that make the case for an acute illness service, distinct from a health service, which wraps around the patient to keep them in good health in the community for longer.

Long-term conditions are a major challenge

Over 15 million people in England currently live with long-term conditions (LTCs). More than two-thirds of the population over 65 years old suffer from one or more LTCs, or multimorbidities. Those with LTCs account for more than 50% of all GP appointments in England and two-thirds of all hospital outpatient appointments and inpatient bed days. This adds up to around 70% of all health and social care expenditure in the UK [1]. Given that this multimorbid group is forecast to be the fastest growing patient group in coming decades, helping those with chronic conditions stay in better health for longer would have the single biggest effect in reducing demand on health-care services.

LTCs are, unsurprisingly, socially patterned (see Fig. 7.1), with the poorest groups having a 60% higher rate of LTCs, whilst the LTCs themselves tend to be about 30% more severe [2]. This group also have the highest levels of workplace absence, health-related benefit payments, and additional needs for informal care from friends and families.

Those with LTCs need us to work together to make the environment one in which it is easy to be healthy, which in turn improves their likelihood of maintaining good health. We also need to ensure that it is easier to access good and appropriate health advice when needed. This would also unlock

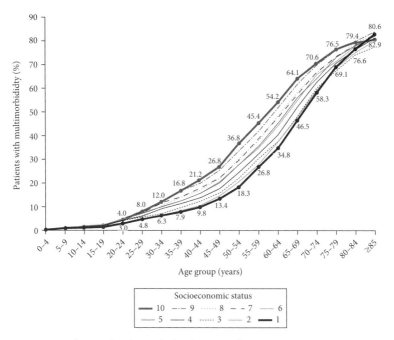

Fig. 7.1 Prevalence of multimorbidity by age and socioeconomic status, Scotland, 2012

years of social health for individuals and whole communities, contributing to redefining the final third of life.

These challenges are not new, but perhaps more pressing now than ever before—healthcare systems are consuming an increasing share of public finances without necessarily improving outcomes, despite the case for the role of good health in prosperity being more compelling than ever. Supporting and empowering individuals to manage their LTCs well would help patients and healthcare systems alike.

Healthcare and the management of LTCs should be delivered through a personalized service that fits the needs of each individual, asking them what they need to stay healthy rather than waiting until they are ill. This is not at odds with the founding principle of the NHS, of universal access to health-care, in fact it furthers it. Equitable access is crucial, but to achieve the same outcome, different population (and risk) groups require different approaches. Yet we still generally pursue an approach that looks at each illness or condition in isolation [1].

Incentives—who pays and who gains?

Incentives and, conversely, disincentives, are some of the most powerful levers for changing the behaviour of individuals, companies, and whole societies. Incentives can be extrinsic motivators and reward actions that result in a defined outcome or metric, or intrinsic motivators, such that the reward is an internally derived satisfaction. When the incentivized outcome does not match the outcome of most concern to the users of a service, that disconnect represents a market failure.

Incentivizing health should be easy because a healthier population (including the health and care workforce themselves) would translate to healthier local and national economies. But in the NHS and many healthcare systems around the world, the payment and commissioning system is activity based, so contributes to a system that inadvertently rewards treating illness, rather than improving health. To make matters more complicated, health services in the UK are delivered through a number of routes, including primary and community care, hospitals, public health under local authorities, and social care, and each of these avenues are commissioned separately, and not all through the NHS, giving each service very little incentive to work together for the total health of the patient.

In an activity based system, the provider of healthcare is paid each time an individual attends a hospital clinic or the emergency department, is admitted to hospital, or has an operation. Hospitals are often paid according to bed occupancy, a sign of illness in a community, rather than bed vacancy rates. Medications are free of charge to individuals in hospitals, yet those same medications have a cost to patients in the community—so we have medications free in illness, costly in health. There is, therefore, a mismatch between the incentives of those providing healthcare and the users of the service.

Providers of healthcare, like any institution, must balance their books, indeed this is how managers of health services are often measured. But under the current system in the UK, for example, 70% of all acute hospital trusts reported financial deficits in the 2018/2019 financial year. This must surely indicate that the system is broken.

There are two major challenges to developing a system that incentivizes health: the disconnect between who pays (generally commissioners or purchasers of healthcare services) and who gains, as the benefits accrue not to the NHS directly but to individuals, their community, and the local economy where the service is delivered; and the time lag between developing a service to promote health and realizing the benefits across a population.

Smoking cessation services provide a useful illustration of the who pays/who gains problem.

In the UK, most public health services were separated from other healthcare services in 2013, moving from the NHS into local government (Local Authorities); smoking cessation services were one such service that transferred to Local Authorities. These services work as part of a whole-system approach to tobacco—the services increase the chance of quitting by up to 53%, which can shift the trajectory of an individual's health and well-being over their lifetime [3]. The benefits, however, are not reaped by those who fund the services. This has serious implications in a world where resources are limited and services and roles are judged by the impact on the bottom line. In this case, the Local Authority pays for the smoking cessation service, but if the service is effective, the reduction in serious healthcare costs will benefit the local clinical commissioning group (NHS), not the Local Authority; the incentives are not aligned.

So it is not surprising that, following the 2013 change, the provision of these services reduced across the country, with some Local Authorities decommissioning the services entirely. At the same time, the healthcare systems responsible for treating the effects of smoking had little or no control over whether, or how, cessation services were delivered. A London-based hospital with patients largely resident across two Local Authorities found that one had decommissioned their smoking cessation service whereas the other had not, so the hospital was only able to offer this service to half of the patients—based not on their risk, nor on their likelihood of responding to the intervention, but based entirely on their postcode.

The complexities of commissioning and delivering healthcare through a number of services and locations contributes to the difficulty of making meaningful change. Since incentives are activity based, they focus attention on short-term delivery and patient numbers, resulting in the perverse situation where hospitals are paid many times more for an outpatient appointment where the patient comes to the hospital than the cost of delivering the same care via a virtual appointment. In many instances, it is better for a patient with an LTC to receive care in the home or local community rather than travel to a perhaps distant hospital, and yet the system does not encourage this patient-centred approach. With this model of commissioning and payments in place and entrenched, there is very little impetus for change, and the long-term benefits that might accrue to society with a total health approach that starts from the individual remain elusive.

When, where, and how we access healthcare

Our individual relationships with the healthcare system are complex, as we have not only different health needs but also different motivators and barriers when seeking and engaging with healthcare services. One size most definitely does not fit all.

If we want to maintain health, then accessing healthcare services needs to be easy. We need to make it easy for each of us to take the measures we need to stay healthy, from vaccinations for ourselves and children to controlling blood pressure and maintaining a healthy weight, especially for those living with LTCs. The will to engage with services whilst not acutely unwell must be greater than the barriers, but accessing services as part of everyday life is often difficult. Where, when, and how we access care when we are acutely unwell with a broken hip or a stroke is clear—the hospital is the best place to be. This is not the case for many of the LTCs that hold us back from day to day life.

In the NHS, access is (generally) equitable even if only delivered via a one-size-fits-all system, so theoretically every member of the public has free access to healthcare. We know, however, that this does not lead to equitable outcomes, nor is it reducing health inequalities. Cancer survival is a striking example. 10,000 deaths could be averted across England over the five years after diagnosis if survival was equitable (see Fig. 7.2). Uptake of cancer services is patchy because people experience their health service differently due to a number of factors, including education, culture, language, and transport options. This is compounded by the fact that coverage, especially in non-emergency scenarios such as breast and cervical screening, is lower in more deprived communities [4].

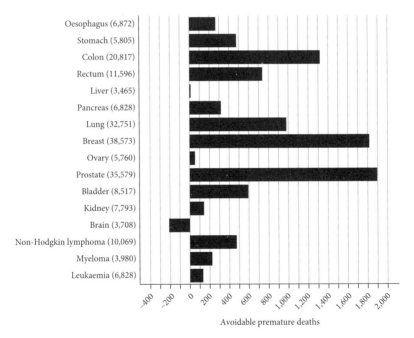

Fig. 7.2 Avoidable premature deaths if survival was equitable among patients diagnosed with cancer in England in 2010

When we access healthcare

We all lead what seem like increasingly busy lives and, despite living longer than ever before, time seems more precious than ever. Across many sectors, our choice of when we access services has increased. Supermarkets and grocery stores, for example, are open outside standard working hours, with supermarkets in the UK now regularly opening as early as 6 am and closing as late as 11 pm seven days a week. Similarly, we can book trains, groceries, other shopping, or holidays at any time of day online, so we have more choice and more options available to us than ever before. This is not the case for healthcare.

According to the British Social Attitudes Survey 2018 [5], the biggest reason for dissatisfaction with the NHS in the UK, in particular in primary care, is the length of time it takes to get an appointment. Indeed, waiting more than two weeks for an appointment with a GP was normal before COVID-19. When we do get an appointment, the choice of the time of day is often restricted. The recent UK National GP Survey found that only 53% of patients are offered a time of day when booking an appointment. This may be because some individuals do not have a preference, or because the issue of concern is so pressing that they can change their schedule to get the earliest possible appointment, it does not make it easy for busy lives.

Core opening hours for primary care services are usually 8 am till 6:30 pm on weekdays, however almost half (46%) of practices are closed at some point during these hours, reducing access further. In fact, almost one in five practices are found to be closed from 3.00 pm onwards at least one afternoon a week. Hence working hours for primary care providers often do not fit with the working lives of their patients, especially in more deprived communities where we find the largest burdens of ill health. Medical and clinical support staff need family friendly practices and flexibility too, so combining their needs with the needs of the public can be hard. Digital can help, as we have seen during the pandemic, both for patients and for clinicians, who are able to work from home if they do not need to see patients in person. But those with acute problems are likely to go to their local hospital instead, increasing the pressure on accident and emergency departments.

Taking the time off work to attend an appointment is not easy or straightforward for many, especially if it means making a choice between lower income in the short term, or lower income in the longer term if the health problem persists. This decision is seen most commonly in deprived communities, where employment is typically precarious and does not include benefits such as sick pay.

We know that providing primary community care services seven days a week and extending opening hours worked in central London when this was put in place. For example, attendances at the local emergency department fell by 8%, with the biggest effect being at the weekends and in those over 65 years old. But in the UK and globally, we are already short of GPs and other primary care practitioners, and given that the shift in attendance patterns was still fairly low, it seems that just extending the present style of service is unlikely to become a game changer in the future.

Nevertheless, we cannot simply do more of the same and expect transformational results; we must be smarter and must do things differently. We need to identify who is best placed to deal with any given healthcare issue, which often may not be a doctor, and use technology to do more with less.

Where we access healthcare

If the choice of when we access healthcare is limited, where we access it is even more restricted. Currently, just 13% of the English population are offered a choice regarding where they access healthcare in the community. A legacy of the founding of the NHS in 1948 was that general practice remained in the private sector whilst hospitals transferred into public ownership. That remains the case for many GP practices, where GPs are the owners of the practice and don't get a salary from the NHS, rather they deliver services commissioned by the NHS and their local authority. This means that GPs are incentivized by the payment system to demonstrate the ongoing need for the same number and size of physical practices and to deliver services at the practice, even though it might be better for the patient to receive that service in the home or elsewhere.

Once again, where we use health services should vary according to the person and their needs. Local pharmacies are easy to access and are starting to be used increasingly to deliver simple vaccination programmes, for instance winter flu vaccination for over 65-year-olds. In winter 2018/19, more than 9,000 community pharmacies (almost 80%) participated in the national NHS flu vaccination programme, providing over 1.4 million flu vaccinations, almost 100,000 more than the previous winter [6].

Why do we not take healthcare to people in supermarkets, at work, at home, or places of leisure? After all, we can order our groceries at work over our lunch break, at home before taking the children to school, or on the train home; comparatively, at every turn as the rest of our lives moves online 24/7, it seems we make it more difficult to engage in healthcare services until we really need it. This has to change.

For many with LTCs, a healthcare setting in the community, or even their own home, is often the best place for their care. Multimorbidity becomes more common with age and multiple complex care needs often require a visit to a health centre. However, healthcare systems generally have a distinct and siloed pathway for each organ, each condition, rather than one approach for the patient, and complex care is generally poorly coordinated. This means that an individual may have to attend separate appointments for each condition that needs treatment. Multiple appointments can be costly, time-consuming, and have serious implications for the individual's ability to work or play as full a role as they want to in families or communities, whilst also increasing the impact of their ill health on their lives.

The ethnographic report of the Richmond Group, aptly titled *Just one thing after another—Living with multiple conditions*, captures the lived experience of living with LTCs [7]. They highlight individuals who had more than 65 medical appointments over the course of a single year and those who, with ten LTCs, attended four different hospitals, six different consultants and two physiotherapists. Such experiences can lead to the individual feeling defined by their health, or ill health. One contributor to the study, with several physical and mental health conditions, commented, 'Deep down it is as if I can't be myself. I am half my health and half me.'

This challenge is not unique to the UK, and there are examples of new models that attempt to address the situation. ChenMed, a healthcare provider in the USA across several States, has developed an approach aimed to simplify the management and control of patients with LTCs. ChenMed take a one-stop shop approach, whereby patients attend one centre to have all of their LTCs addressed in just one visit. This polyclinic approach has generalists and specialists on site, along with a dispensing pharmacy. They take a holistic approach to the patient's care, with one manager responsible for overseeing the coordination of their care, and provide transport if required to help the individual attend their monthly appointment.

Perhaps unsurprisingly, the evidence suggests this approach works. Chenmed found both improved patient outcomes, including reductions in common risk factors such as cholesterol, as well as benefits to the healthcare providers, seen in a reduction in hospitalization rates of 18% and readmissions by 70%. Probably the most encouraging feature is that they achieved these in a population that is predominantly covered by Medicare, typically older and poorer populations who for decades have had the worst health outcomes. This is just one example, and a similar approach is being trialled in England through the NHS Vanguard programmes, especially for the elderly living in care homes.

How we access healthcare

How all of us access goods and services has changed dramatically over the past decade. Technology has transformed our experience and daily life, but healthcare has not kept up, indeed access to healthcare in the UK has stagnated or even reduced over the last decade.

In 2012, 78% of the population reported it being easy to get through to healthcare services by telephone [8]. That figure had declined to 68% in 2017. Just under 9% of us booked our healthcare appointments online in 2017, up just one percentage point over the last three years, 16% order repeat prescriptions online and only 4% of us access our medical records online. We have allowed technology and the possibilities it offers to by-pass healthcare or, where there are good ideas or examples, it has been almost impossible to scale them across the NHS.

The role of power and control in incentivizing health

For most of us, even if we do not recognize it, control or agency is the most important dimension of our lives. The degree to which we feel in control over our work patterns, control over the lives we lead and the people we spend time with, or how and when we see a doctor, is a direct function of the degree to which we are in control of the way that experience unfolds. The Whitehall Study infamously found that those in the lower rungs of the civil service, who had much less control over their work patterns and day-to-day lives, suffered three times higher death rates than the most senior civil servants [9].

Experiencing ill health leaves a sense of lack of control. We do not choose when we become ill, and feel we do not know what is happening to us or what is coming next. Those with LTCs often feel they are unable to plan life normally, in case their health worsens, or because of their multiple medical appointments. This can define an individual and remove their sense of independence and control of day-to-day life. As one contributor to the Richmond Group study on living with LTCs told them: 'It is frustrating that no matter how self-controlled I am, my resistance to insulin will grow and there's nothing I can do to stop that.' This woman has type 1 diabetes and monitors her glucose levels with a sensor, using the information to determine the amount of insulin she requires in her regular injections. The impact on her and her daily life could be reduced if she were fitted with an insulin pump that automatically titrated her insulin according to her glucose levels.

Traditionally, doctors took all the decisions about treatment and care, but increasingly the decision is shared between the patient and the doctor. This has not, however, translated into shared and empowered control of LTCs. Information can be empowering and increase the sense of control, but it has to be actionable, as information alone can also have the opposite effect and contribute to lower feelings of control.

Information about health and health behaviours can come from many sources. Mass media campaigns have been used for decades to inform the population in the hope of changing behaviour. The five-a-day fruit and vegetables campaign has been used in the UK, USA, and many other countries with mixed results. Recognition and understanding of the five-a-day message, that eating five or more portions of fruit and vegetables a day is good for health, is high. But that recognition has not translated into large and sustained changes in behaviour.

Time and time again we see that information alone cannot help overcome the three As—accessibility, affordability and availability—whilst the marketing budget of companies promoting less healthy foods dwarfs the spend on information campaigns. In 2017 in the UK, over £300 million was spent advertising soft drinks, confectionary, and sweet snacks compared to just £16 million advertising fruits and vegetables [10].

Similar challenges have emerged around an increasingly understood driver of our health, genetics. Genomic screening has become more available and cheaper. We can now buy a readout of our entire genome online that will identify any known mutations which may predispose us to a given disease. But providing related information, such as having an increased risk of obesity or heart disease, in and of itself has little effect on changing behaviour to mitigate that risk. Indeed, it can leave individuals feeling more disempowered. As one contributor to the Richmond Group study reflected, 'You look at the medical report and think what the heck does that mean, so it is easier to wait and see the GP who can explain it in layman's terms.' Combining information about a risk with actionable information as to how to reduce that risk is much more likely to work and be sustainable. The extra challenge, though, is having enough clinicians with enough time to interpret the information and explain the options.

From activities to outcomes: a way to make health and prevention pay for everyone

There have been many efforts to identify and implement alternative payment systems that incentivize monitoring or improving the health of the patient, rather than treatment activity alone. Many agree with the idea of having a healthcare system that focuses upon delivering the best outcomes to those using the system; outcomes- or value-based commissioning aims to do just that. Put simply, outcomes-based commissioning is an approach to the funding of healthcare services based on the outcome of the patient that puts individuals at the centre of the commissioning process.

In theory, this approach incentivizes all involved in the care of a patient to achieve the best outcomes for that patient whether they are in their home, the community, social care, or hospital. The payment is tied to the health of the patient and shared across those who contribute to it, rather than just paying each provider at each stage of care. Outcomes-based commissioning aims to encourage providers across the healthcare sector to work together on the outcomes that matter most to people—be that keeping people independent and in their own home for longer, controlling their LTCs so they can participate in day-to-day life, or engaging with healthcare services early to prevent a minor condition worsening. The pooling of these risks and rewards could contribute to a shift in focus on preventative and self-care services and foster a more innovative ecosystem that helps to identify solutions for some of the biggest challenges of today, such as frailty and multimorbidity, in a researching and learning system in which all are incentivized.

Healthcare company Kaiser Permanente harnesses this approach to ensure that the health of the individual has priority. It is the largest non-profit health plan provider in the US and is globally renowned for effectively integrating healthcare services to deliver cutting edge patient care for more than 12 million people. Through coordinating care across primary and secondary care with community assets such as pharmacies, Kaiser Permanente has united their group around delivering care that aims to keep each individual as healthy as possible.

Users of the service cite accessing and receiving care to be easier than in previous health plans, with much of this achieved with the help and support of technology and data analytics. Any clinician that a patient encounters in Kaiser Permanente, for example, has access to their comprehensive electronic health record (via KP HealthConnect), which updates in real-time whether in the community or a hospital.

Kaiser Permanente prioritizes prevention with impressive results— achieving a reduction in smoking prevalence of 25% in their users in California compared to just 7.5% across the state more generally—and they are committed to monitoring and comparing the health of individuals with LTCs using data registries that keep clinicians regularly informed.

Preventative care pays. This matters in the increasingly expensive health sector with increasingly expensive medical problems. One example from Kaiser Permanente is their Collaborative Cardiac Care Service for patients who have suffered heart attacks. The patients are assigned a nurse manager as soon as they arrive in the hospital, who encourages them to participate in follow-up services, including cardiac rehabilitation and psychological support as well as risk-factor reduction programmes such as smoking cessation. The coordination of care continues once the patient leaves hospital, with local clinical pharmacists taking on the role, monitoring their progress and adjusting the programmes accordingly. Introduced over 10 years ago, this programme has had substantial impact—increasing the proportion of patients with their cholesterol controlled by three-fold, reducing death rates by a huge 73%, and generating $30 million savings each year for the provider; a healthier population saves lives and money [11,12].

There are challenges to designing a system like this and then making it happen, but none are insurmountable. Often groups within healthcare fear the risk of losing status and control, not seeing how this would ease the pressure on their services. The use of high-dimensional data analytics incorporating health risks and lived patient experiences is key, as are actuarial approaches to the pooling of risk. We see growing examples of such cross-sector learning within health, but for preventative systems to flourish this needs leadership, nationally and locally, to make the case as to why health, rather than illness, is an opportunity for all.

Putting health back into healthcare

Our current healthcare system is creaking, unable to adequately meet the demand from patients and our ageing and multimorbid population. Our NHS has shown to have little resilience when COVID-19 hit and it did no better than European neighbours when faced with the pandemic.

But there is cause for optimism. The pandemic has demonstrated that, whilst the NHS has been trying to both treat illness and deliver health, the incentives, structures, and skills required are very different. We recognize that we need an illness system that is the best in class, resilient to the unexpected such as COVID-19, but that this same system will not deliver the healthy living dividend that will unlock prosperity, happiness, and fairness across communities and nations. We need to think differently.

A healthcare system that keeps us independent in our own homes for longer focusing on what matters to us is actually closer than ever. In England, even before COVID-19 struck, 'GP at hand', a digital-first primary care service operated by Babylon, had seen a dramatic influx of patients to the service since its introduction. Patients liked the technology and it was a first for the UK, but transferring to Babylon negatively affected the funding of their original GPs. With an estimated 90% of primary care consultations becoming 'digital first' during the first wave of the pandemic, we have an opportunity to embed this approach more widely, remembering that, as with all emerging technologies, we must balance patient choice with safety and data protection.

A new Health Index: what gets measured, gets managed

If we continue to measure illness, we can expect to have healthcare systems focused on illness when actually everyone wants health. This has historical roots—in the early 20th century, water, sanitation, and housing improvements contributed to improving health while healthcare systems were largely judged by illness treatment. Now, in the 21st century post COVID-19, health and equity must be at the heart of how our systems, and the leaders who operate them, are measured and judged. Healthcare systems have a dual role going forward; to treat illness and to deliver total health.

In the UK, a composite Health Index is being developed by the Office for National Statistics (ONS) to sit alongside GDP. We introduced the concept in the Chief Medical Officer's independent 2018 annual report. The idea of the Health Index is rooted in repositioning total health as an asset to a nation, rather than ill health being a drain. Current measures keep us unable to identify the key determinants of total health, nor flag and intervene before it is too late because the focus has been on traditional outcome measures such as life expectancy. The Health Index instead recognizes total health to be an opportunity for economic prosperity and happiness. As we look to rebuild society post-COVID-19, the index will capture the complex factors that represent our stock of total health and track communities' and the nation's progress to a healthier future.

Specifically, the proposed Composite Health Index has three layers: health outcomes such as infant mortality and cancer survival; modifiable risk factors such as the prevalence of overweight, obesity, and smoking; and the social and economic determinants of health, such as the percentage of the population living in relative poverty, in insecure employment or with access to green spaces. Importantly, health inequalities would be captured at each level.

The ONS have grouped these under three domains—Healthy People, Healthy Lives, Healthy Places. Through putting health, and importantly equitable health, at the heart of government planning and monitoring, we believe this can incentivize the development of policies that promote health and equity, and deliver dividends for all.

Population Health Management

Coupled with the concept of a Health Index, there is now growing interest in Population Health Management (PHM) as an opportunity to redress the balance between health and illness services. PHM is the idea that we shift health services from thinking only about individual diseases and isolated interventions to considering how best to keep whole groups, thus for instance populations with LTCs, living well for longer.

Epidemiology is the study of disease patterns by time, place, and person— it describes the problem— whilst PHM aims to not only understand the problem, but also to examine the complex and multidimensional drivers of health and ultimately design more collaborative and integrated services that put health first. PHM is gaining traction, partly because we all know a more joined-up approach is required. Indeed, NHS England has prioritized PHM as a key approach as they push for care services to become more integrated.

In addition, PHM helps us to better understand the relationship between interventions now and the time lag before the benefits are realized. For instance, a cancer screening programme must be paid for now, but it will only bear fruit later in the form of increased survival rates due to early diagnosis, cheaper treatments as fewer interventions are required, and the fact that those detected and treated early will remain active at work and in the community for longer. It is currently seen to be very hard to justify a budget now that can only be properly reviewed in 20 or 30 years' time to see if it was money well spent.

Still in its relative infancy, PHM has perhaps more alternative definitions and theoretical frameworks than worked examples implemented in practice. There are international examples, however, such as the Kaiser Permanente illustration described earlier. A health system fit for the 21st century must harness the core aspects of PHM.

Time to align incentives and total health

To accept the need for change and coordinated but parallel approaches for illness and health systems will need innovative and brave leadership. Many of our proposed solutions are not new, and there are examples of good practice, generally in isolated places. Aligning incentives around the health of individuals and populations should be straight forward, but we need to explore who should fund these and who, alongside the individual, should benefit.

It has become increasingly popular in health to describe the complexities of the drivers of our health and the broad health system itself, yet meaningful interventions that can be implemented tomorrow have been put in place too rarely. The blockers include funding flows, structures, process, heavy bureaucracy, power struggles, and the lack of a unified vision around which to come together.

But we have an opportunity. The contrast of the pre-COVID-19 NHS with now is dramatic. National data on PPE, bed vacancies, staffing, and drugs is being used to inform day-to-day decisions. It has also become much easier to order repeat prescriptions, by emailing the GP and receiving a text from the pharmacy when it is ready to collect, with home delivery options for those who need it.

The healthcare system has a great number of actors. From those delivering care on the front line—doctors, nurses, care assistants, and other key workers—to those in policy, and from those commissioning (or buying) the care we receive to the life science industry providing new medications, devices, and technologies. Throughout this chapter, however, we have outlined that despite the advances of modern medicine helping us all live longer, the healthcare system is no longer working for us—citizens and patients—to live in good health for longer. At each turn it is easier for us as citizens and our healthcare workers not to engage pre-emptively in our health or to give us control over our LTCs so we can get on and enjoy our lives.

As we look to the future we should remember why the NHS was established, who our healthcare systems serve, and how we can best serve those populations. We must ensure they are designed and incentivized to deliver good health to all.

References

1. Department of Health. *Long-term conditions compendium of Information: Third edition*. Department of Health and Social Care. 2012.
2. The King's Fund Time to think differently. Long terms conditions and multi-morbidity. The King's Fund. 2013. https://www.kingsfund.org.uk/projects/time-think-differently/trends-disease-and-disability-long-term-conditions-multi-morbidity
3. Bauld L, Bell K, McCullough L, Richardson L, Greaves L. The effectiveness of NHS smoking cessation services: a systematic review. *J Public Health (Oxf)*. 2010;32(1):71–82. doi:10.1093/pubmed/fdp074
4. Douglas E, Waller J, Duffy SW, Wardle J. Socioeconomic inequalities in breast and cervical screening coverage in England: are we closing the gap? *J Med Screen*. 2016 Jun;23(2):98–103. doi: 10.1177/0969141315600192. Epub 2015 Sep 16. PMID: 26377810; PMCID: PMC4855247.
5. Phillips D, Curtice J, Phillips M, Perry J. (eds.) *British Social Attitudes: The 35th Report*. London: The National Centre for Social Research. 2018.
6. Pharmaceutical Services Negotiating Committee. Flu vaccination data for 2018/2019. Accessed: https://psnc.org.uk/services-commissioning/advanced-services/flu-vaccination-service/flu-vaccination-statistics/flu-vaccination-data-for-2018-19/
7. The Richmond Group of Charities. *'Just one thing after another': Living with multiple conditions*. A report from the taskforce on multiple conditions. October 2018: https://richmondgroupofcharities.org.uk/sites/default/files/final_just_one_thing_after_another_report_-_singles.pdf
8. Wellings D, Baird B. Patient experience of GP surgeries: it's getting in that's the problem. The King's Fund. July 2017: https://www.kingsfund.org.uk/blog/2017/07/patient-experience-gp-surgeries-its-getting-thats-problem
9. Marmot M, Rose G, Shipley M, Hamilton P. Employment grade and coronary heart disease in British civil servants. Journal of Epidemiology and Community Health. 1978;**32** (4):244–49. doi:10.1136/jech.32.4.244. PMC 1060958. PMID 744814.
10. The Food Foundation. *The Broken Plate*. 2019.

11. Sandhoff B, Kuca S, Rasmussen J, Merenich J. Collaborative cardiac care service: a multidisciplinary approach to caring for patients with coronary artery disease. *Perm J*. 2008;12(3):4–11. doi:10.7812/tpp/08-007

12. Mckinsey. What health systems can learn from Kaiser Permanente; an interview with Hal Wolf. *Health International Number 8*. 2009: https://www.mckinsey.com/~/media/mckinsey/dotcom/client_service/Healthcare%20Systems%20and%20Services/Health%20International/HI08_Kaiser_Permanente.ashx

8
The promise of technology

Healthcare owes much of its success to technology, from penicillin, aspirin, and blood transfusions to transplantation, monoclonal antibodies, genomics, modern imaging, and surgery. Today, emerging and digital technologies—the fourth industrial revolution—have the potential to transform health and care services, making it better and easier for staff and patients, but unfortunately public health and healthcare are yet to participate fully in the digital era. Public services as a whole lag way behind other sectors, let alone their users, the public. To drive change, both users of healthcare and those working in it must demand better and play their part in making it happen, through embracing digital approaches and managing their introduction into use.

In this chapter, we focus on how technology can contribute to the three pillars of health we discuss throughout this book by: helping the healthcare system to do more with less; empowering individuals with chronic conditions to live well for longer; and providing the tools to make populations healthier in the 21st century.

Enabling clinicians to deliver the best care to patients

By augmenting human performance, AI has the potential to mark-edly improve productivity, efficiency, workflow, accuracy and speed, both for [physicians] and for patients . . . What I'm most excited about is using the future to bring back the past: to restore the care in healthcare.

Eric Topol, director and founder of Scripps Research Translational Institute

One of the biggest challenges facing the delivery of healthcare globally is that systems are simply not able to keep pace with the rising complexity and volume of need from their expanding and ageing populations. Artificial intelligence (AI) has great potential to transform the delivery of healthcare

Whose Health Is It, Anyway? Dame Sally C. Davies and Jonathan Pearson-Stuttard, Oxford University Press (2021).
© Oxford University Press. DOI: 10.1093/oso/9780198863458.003.0008

and mitigate this. Most of what is often referred to as 'AI' across healthcare is actually machine learning (ML). ML is based on pattern recognition using deep learning algorithms that are trained to perform specific tasks by extracting patterns and information from a set of data without humans programming how to achieve this. It is not surprising therefore, that some of the most promising early work in healthcare has been in imaging and digital pathology. The potential uses, however, are much broader; from enabling clinicians to have much more personalized detail of a patient's treatment needs and likely prognosis, to the development of new drugs. ML offers great promise in a profession and industry where having the right information at the right time is key.

As with other sectors, the potential of automation has led some within the healthcare workforce to worry about their job security. However, as Mark Britnell, chairman of KPMG healthcare, wrote recently, 'our workforce is already woefully short; we have too few doctors and nurses to provide the care need for our population now' [1]. This gap is only forecast to worsen, with projections suggesting the world will be five million doctors short by 2030 [2]. Far from replacing the need for doctors and nurses, AI and other emerging technologies could provide much-needed support and relief to an already overstretched workforce.

The great potential of ML in healthcare has been discussed in detail in other books so we briefly give three illustrative examples to show how ML could help the delivery of care, free up time, and help move healthcare from a focus on illness to delivering total health. These examples highlight that coalescing around shared values between partners and patients can bring innovations to healthcare much faster than if the health system continues to work siloed from what is going on in the rest of the world around us.

Prioritizing interventions

Prioritizing which patient needs to be seen first is a perennial challenge for clinicians on a busy ward round. All patients in hospital need support, but who will deteriorate soonest without attention and who could be discharged back home today if their medications are ready? In the NHS, one in ten patients suffers some form of avoidable harm whilst in hospital [3]. So can we get the patient home or pick up problems early? Through identifying the early signs of deterioration in health we are already seeing the potential of AI in supporting clinicians to tackle this.

The Streams app developed by Deepmind has been piloted in patients with acute kidney injury (AKI) at the Royal Free Hospital in London over the last couple of years. AKI affects up to approximately 15% of all hospital admissions in England, with adverse consequences for the patient and substantial costs to the hospital. The Streams app monitors real-time data relevant to AKI, interprets the data, and provides this information to clinicians. The trial found that just 3% of AKI cases were missed by the Streams technology compared to 12% before the technology was implemented. Streams also helped prioritize the most urgent cases, resulting in them being reviewed quicker; the evaluation found that Streams enabled an expert to assess each and every AKI patient within 15 minutes at any time of the day. And the roll-out of this technology was found to reduce the average healthcare cost per patient by more than £2,000.

Improving speed and accuracy of diagnosis

If clinicians come to the right diagnosis quickly, patients can get the best care without delay; this can also mean fewer invasive tests and less time in hospital. A recent study at Massachusetts Institute of Technology, for example, found that ML could help predict whether breast lesions on breast imaging scans traditionally read as high risk are in fact truly cancerous or actually benign. The authors found this technology reduced unnecessary procedures by a third, and any interventions needed could take place more quickly.

A delay in accurate diagnosis can cost lives or result in permanent injury or disability. Both age and diabetes are leading causes of common eye conditions such as macular degeneration. The Moorfields Eye Hospital in London has seen a dramatic increase in the number of patients requiring eye scans as our population gets older and diabetes becomes more common. The rising numbers means that there can be a delay in reading and diagnosing a scan, and consequently a delay in beginning the appropriate treatment. This can have devastating consequences for patients as, until an eye scan has been performed and interpreted by a trained ophthalmologist, it is not clear whether a patient requires surgery to prevent sight-loss or not.

Moorfields collaborated with Deepmind to see whether using ML could help to improve the speed at which patients with diseases that threatened their sight, particularly age-related macular degeneration, could be diagnosed without any loss of accuracy. The ML system 'learned' by analysing thousands of historical optical coherence tomography (OCT) scans and

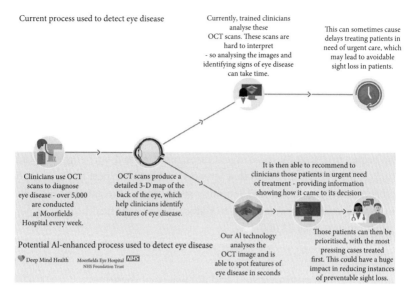

Current process used to detect eye disease

Currently, trained clinicians analyse these OCT scans. These scans are hard to interpret - so analysing the images and identifying signs of eye disease can take time.

This can sometimes cause delays treating patients in need of urgent care, which may lead to avoidable sight loss in patients.

Clinicians use OCT scans to diagnose eye disease - over 5,000 are conducted at Moorfields Hospital every week.

OCT scans produce a detailed 3-D map of the back of the eye, which help clinicians identify features of eye disease.

It is then able to recommend to clinicians those patients in urgent need of treatment - providing information showing how it came to its decision

Potential AI-enhanced process used to detect eye disease

Deep Mind Health   Moorfields Eye Hospital *NHS* NHS Foundation Trust

Our AI technology analyses the OCT image and is able to spot features of eye disease in seconds

Those patients can then be prioritised, with the most pressing cases treated first. This could have a huge impact in reducing instances of preventable sight loss.

Fig. 8.1 Current process vs potential AI-enhanced process to detect eye disease

Reproduced from Davies SC, Annual Report of the Chief Medical Officer, 2018. Health 2040 – Better Health Within Reach, Copyright (2018), Department of Health and Social Care. Reproduced under the Open Government Licence v3.0. Original source: Reproduced from Suleyman M, A Major Milestone for the Treatment of Eye Disease, Copyright (2018), Deepmind.

medical reports to identify what is normal and the features of eye disease, and then made recommendations regarding the most appropriate referral for the conditions identified (see Fig. 8.1). The team found that the ML system made the correct referral recommendation more than 94% of the time, which matched the performance of their expert clinicians. Importantly, this process of interpreting and providing a recommendation was done in approximately one minute, compared to the three hours required by the expert clinician [4]. Moreover, the tool can be used successfully on digital scans sent via the web, thus helping patients remotely, wherever they are.

Using resources efficiently and effectively

Every second the doctor is not seeing patients is wasted time. Doctors already spend roughly 40 percent of their day documenting and doing other administrative tasks. To waste the other 50 to

60 percent of your day traveling between patients is a 50 to 60 per-
cent reduction in efficiency. Short of teleportation, the doctor house
call will always be an irresponsibly massive reduction in primary
care efficiency.

Dr. Jay Parkinson, Founder and Chief Medical Officer, Sherpaa

As much as 50% of clinicians' time is spent simply entering data or writing notes. The data itself is invaluable to the patient's treatment and continuity of care, but could also be used to inform risk profiles and trajectories and wider research—but sadly currently much of this data is not used to improve population-wide patient care.

The data recording process is also a source of errors; ML, again, promises solutions. Natural Language Processing, whereby computers process and analyse large amounts of language data, is a practical tool that could both reduce medical errors and free up clinicians' time to focus on interacting with and treating patients. Natural Language Processing offers a wide range of other potential opportunities, from improving medication adherence to providing reminders and organizing transportation for medical appointments.

Identifying the most appropriate care, with the most appropriate clinician, at the most appropriate time and appropriate place for each patient is a real challenge. Getting this wrong costs extra time and money for already stretched healthcare services, and risks delay to care which has knock-on effects on the patient's prognosis. Efforts to improve triaging processes include NHS 111 in England, which replaced the previous system, NHS Direct. NHS 111 is a medical helpline, via telephone and online, for urgent but not life-threatening health issues. It acts as a triage system for less severe health issues and to reduce demand on emergency ambulance services.

Chatbots, technologies that use Natural Language Processing to interact with users, can synthesize spoken language, data from past history, and real-time measurements such as blood pressure and heart rate to aid this. AI has the capability to advise clinicians, or administrative staff, which patients need an appointment and with whom, the urgency, and also the modality (telephone, video, or face to face). This technology continues to develop, but it is vital that it is accurate as the stakes are so high—an algorithm mistakenly deeming a patient to have heartburn, rather than a potentially fatal heart attack, would not be acceptable.

Getting these technologies into use to help patients and clinicians brings new challenges. Many interventions in the past were static—they could be assessed in a randomized controlled trial and, if effective, rolled out in the knowledge that they would not change. ML and other emerging technologies learn and evolve. Their uses range from booking appointments to suggesting treatments, so a tailored approach is required to assess effectiveness and safety, and this has to be proportionate to what the technology is doing.

Wearables and digital therapeutics could put choice and control back into the hands of citizens

Wearable technologies contribute through enabling better control, they can help people adopt healthy lifestyles, and can improve the health of individuals living with long-term conditions (LTCs). Wearables can also reset the balance of power in managing LTCs between the individual and their own health, and also between the patient and the doctor.

The goal for tackling LTCs is to manage them sufficiently well so that the risk of complications, hospitalization, and early death are minimized, allowing patients to live a normal, uninterrupted life as far as possible. One of the biggest challenges in achieving this has been that there are often few signs that an individual's health is deteriorating until it is too late. Accurate monitoring usually requires frequent trips to the doctor or nurse and often multiple visits for difference LTCs. Wearable technologies could not only make this monitoring easier in real time, but also interpret the reading for the patient and flag concerns to the clinical team early enough to allow prevention. Monitoring blood sugar levels in those with diabetes is a prime example; early identification of blood sugars going too low or too high can help prevent the patient from becoming unwell and requiring hospitalization.

Two significant scientific and technological advances are converging. Progress in material sciences is enabling us to monitor more and more clinical biomarkers in smaller and less invasive devices. Novel biosensors that use such innovations can be the size of a sticking plaster. Examples include patches prototyped by the University of California San Diego, where complex circuitry is incorporated into a flexible and breathable wearable that provides ongoing monitoring of glucose levels in patients with diabetes.

As patients with diabetes can expect a multitude of complications, such as heart attacks, stroke and renal disease, while diabetes is also associated with increased risk of musculoskeletal or mental health conditions, and much more, real-time glucose monitoring, through sweat for example, could be a game changer. Importantly, these technologies are falling dramatically in cost, meaning that they could become affordable to consumers and health-care providers around the world.

Another promising approach is pathogen detection through breath analyses. Integrating these, other health data, and additional citizen-generated data (e.g. local levels of air pollution) could give a more real-time holistic risk trajectory for a particular individual and then help to ensure they receive the best care.

In almost every other sector, digitization has led to an explosion of choice, transparency, and re-balancing of markets around consumer preference and ease. There are a few examples of the early stages of this in health—for instance health insurers providing incentives such as free coffee if individuals walk 10,000 steps each day, and reduced premiums for attending groups or taking exercise. But this is not systematic and the important thing is to tie the behaviour and incentives to health outcomes.

In the world of retail banking, we log in on smartphones to check our balance, deposits, and payments, and to pay bills. Importantly we can do this at any time of day from anywhere. This allows real-time, dynamic monitoring of our money and, if our account drops into deficit, an automated message informs us by text and/or email. In fact, many banks now offer other automated alerts—a text message every time the account is used, or if certain thresholds on the account are crossed. Our health is a commodity too, yet currently we generally only monitor it at fixed time points, rarely in real-time and often when our health 'balance' has been in the red for some time and maybe even irreversibly.

> MS impairs the ability to walk for many people with MS, yet we only assess walking ability in the limited time a patient is in the doctor's office. Consumer devices can measure number of steps, distance walked, and sleep quality on a continuous basis in a person's home environment. These data could provide potentially important information to supplement office visit exams.
>
> Dr. Richard Rudick, VP of Value Based Medicine, Biogen

In the Chief Medical Officer's 2018 annual report, Professor Mihaela van der Schaar and colleagues introduced the concept of an 'Electronic Health Engine' [5]. Traditional electronic health records are static, they contain information that was inputted into the system in the past, usually during specific health consultations, and thus provide an out-dated and non-comprehensive view of our past health. In future, a dynamic platform that integrates information and data from wearables that is not just about our ill health, but also about the drivers of total health, would revolutionize patient experience, health outcomes, and much more.

The increasing wealth of information about our health risks combined with computing power and advances in ML, mean that an individualized, condition-specific health trajectory that dynamically integrates data inputs is within reach. Not only should such a system be able to automate notifications to alert either us or our clinicians that (preventative) action should be taken, but it would also provide a much more holistic view of our risk, and how we can change this for the better. This would be genuinely personalized prevention and maintenance of our total health. It could also mean large savings for healthcare providers.

There are, of course, challenges to overcome regarding data sharing and privacy. Our data is valuable, and plenty of technology companies already know and exploit this, but whose data is it? We must find a balance whereby we all see a data dividend personally and through better services and health for all.

We know that, with transparency and true engagement, patients and families understand and appreciate the benefits to themselves and others of health data, suitably anonymized, being analysed at group and population level. One successful example is the sharing of whole genome data and clinical features from patients with rare diseases, their families, and patients with cancer in the NHS 100,000 Whole Genome Project run by Genomics England. The discourse regarding technology and technology based companies though, has generally focused not on these positive stories but rather on the negatives, such as the Cambridge Analytica scandal, when data about individuals was sold and used for purposes the individual was unaware of and did not consent to.

AI more broadly, not just ML, could indeed transform the delivery of healthcare for all, conversely, without good planning it could in fact worsen health inequalities and erode public trust in doctors and nurses, currently the most trusted professions in the UK. Recent research by Future Advocacy has found the public's willingness to trust algorithms depend upon answers to certain questions: What is the success rate of the AI? Where does the AI come from, who developed it? What kind of data was the AI trained on? Will the AI work well for me, if I am a member of a minority group? All reasonable questions that need answering through systematic and inclusive research approaches.

Some technologies not only promote healthy behaviours but also create a social network and gamify being healthy. Just as obesity is associated with family and social networks, healthy behaviours can be too. Strava is a social fitness network that uses the GPS of the user to track exercise, particularly cycling and running. Users can plan and share their cycling and running routes, distances, speeds, and frequency with their network. Many users cite the technology being free to use as one of the key reasons behind its success, that their friends and family also use it, and that it harnesses peer-pressure for good—an extra incentive to get out on that morning run even when the weather is wet and windy. This has a positive effect on physical, mental, and social health.

Citizen generated data such as that captured by Strava is not currently routinely captured within our health records, but could be useful for calculating our future health risks and for considering preventive measures.

Predictive prevention—new tools for public health

An ounce of prevention is worth a pound of cure.

Benjamin Franklin

One of the key benefits of technology is the ability to rapidly analyse large amounts of data, and the flow of data from various sources that informs health and healthcare is growing all the time. We generally see three groups of data capturing our health and drivers of health: patient-generated data capturing clinical metrics in and out of the hospital; public and population data on risk factors such as pollution and smoking prevalence; and citizen-generated data through smart phones and other devices that capture individual lifestyle data such as number of steps or cycling patterns. Advances in computing power and ML-based methods make prevention using these datasets more possible today than ever before. Technologies that utilize AI could facilitate embedding a truly preventative healthcare system.

Our understanding of the multiple complex drivers of our total health and specific conditions or clusters of conditions, such as cardiovascular disease, is developing alongside the ability to use ML to incorporate a large number of wide-ranging data types and sources, including formal medical records and citizen-generated data capturing social and even commercial drivers of health. This in turn takes us beyond traditional statistical methods and allows more accurate stratification of risk for individuals and populations, so that the most effective interventions can be targeted towards those most in need, and interventions that will not work or that are not needed can be avoided. This will lead to the mainstream use of intelligent 'predict and prevent' services.

Predictive analytics can be applied to a wide range of areas across healthcare. Whilst many of the applications will be aimed at precise information in order to intervene more specifically, and often earlier, in the course of a disease, there are several areas where harnessing predictive analytics could actually lead to less, rather than more, healthcare. Screening programmes for several common cancers, for example, currently tend to adopt a one-size-fits-all approach whereby screening is carried out for every individual at a fixed interval, for example three-yearly for breast cancer screening in women aged 50-70 years in the UK. We know however, that the risk of breast cancer is not equal within the population, so there will be those for whom three-yearly tests are an unnecessarily frequent invasive procedure and costly, and others at an increased risk, perhaps because of the presence of one or several known genetic mutations, who are likely to benefit from more frequent and targeted screening.

Risk stratification tools, such as QRISK for cardiovascular disease (CVD), have been used for many years [6]. QRISK uses a range of risk factors including age, blood pressure, cholesterol, body mass index, ethnicity, and socio-economic deprivation, as well as several other health co-morbidities such as chronic kidney disease and diabetes. A clinician puts in the patient's values for this wide range of factors to produce a QRISK score—that is the percentage chance of a CVD event over the next ten years. An individual QRISK above ten prompts the clinician to consider prescribing preventative medicine, such as statins, to reduce cholesterol levels.

The QRISK algorithm is updated annually to include additional risk factors, for instance ethnicity and socio-economic deprivation were added in the second iteration in an attempt to reduce health inequalities. An individual, user-friendly online-tool has also been developed. This tool is, however, largely static, with the rules of the algorithm programmed in advance, leading to an inflexible process that is difficult to update. The associations are often crude too, do not account for differences in risk of CVD according to population sub-group, and also take one disease in isolation despite this being increasingly rare in practice.

Polygenic risk scores based on genome scans have been found to outperform QRISK, and ML methods could transform static, general tools like these into real-time and personalized tools that deliver much better health dividends by using the increasingly available broader data sets and hence transform these predictive processes. The wider datasets include genomic data quantifying susceptibility or protection from several common conditions to citizen-generated data capturing physical activity, sedentary time, and sleep time—and enabling dynamic risk prediction that updates in real-time according to lifestyle and behaviour.

Diabetes is a good example of how this approach might benefit sufferers. Diabetes is a very varied disease, both in how it manifests and also the trajectory of the disease, and has become increasingly prevalent globally, alongside the rise in obesity. It is crippling healthcare systems and hampering the lives of millions through disability and their inability to lead normal lives. Individuals living with diabetes are, like those without diabetes, living longer than ever before, but with a larger portion of life lived in poor health. This longevity has increased and diversified the conditions which those living with diabetes suffer from, extending to cancers, common infections, liver disease, and dementias as well as vascular conditions [7]. A similar pattern of broad sequelae is now emerging in those living with obesity.

ML approaches have the potential to tailor diabetes prevention and treatment efforts more specifically to individuals. Emerging evidence combining ML methods with a wider set of mixed datasets on genetics, anti-pancreas antibodies, blood measurement, body mass index, and much more, has suggested diabetes can be grouped more specifically than the standard categorization of type 1 (insulin dependent) and type 2 (non-insulin dependent). Scientists in Sweden have proposed five clusters with differences in disease progression and future development of complications [8]:

- Cluster 1 generally experience onset of disease early in life, are generally not overweight or obese but have poor glucose control and the presence of antibodies that destroy the cells in the pancreas that produce insulin.
- Cluster 2 have similar characteristics to those in cluster 1 but without the pancreas-destroying antibodies.
- Cluster 3 are generally obese with poor metabolic control and insulin resistance (when cells in muscles, fat and liver become less sensitive to insulin hence less sugar is taken from the blood into cells).
- Cluster 4 are generally obese, but without insulin resistance and with a much milder form of diabetes.
- Cluster 5 are characterized as being older and obesity being less dominant, age-related diabetes, with only modest metabolic derangements.

Clearly, better definitions and diagnosis can lead to better prevention, treatment, and outcomes. The pace of scientific advances in our understanding of diabetes combined with AI offers real hope in personalizing preventative monitoring, both to keep people in good health for longer and to avoid unnecessary testing and interventions where they will not be useful to a particular individual.

Simulated populations for simulated futures

Randomized controlled trials (RCTs) have long been seen as the gold standard in establishing causality and effectiveness within health. RCTs are, however, expensive, prolonged, and can be impractical or unethical for some population health issues, such as smoke-free legislation, or how planning legislation could affect pollution levels in cities and the subsequent health effects. Advances in data science have great potential to make it easier for policymakers to visualize the potential effects of these and other policies to inform actions.

'In silico medicine' describes the use of computer simulation to model and visualize health issues in a virtual environment. Simulation modelling can be embedded across policy and decision making—as is frequently done in economics and meteorology but rarely so in health. As with any forecasting, simulation modelling is imperfect and cannot provide absolute certainty when looking to the future, but it is able to produce estimates of the potential effects upon health, costs, and inequalities of a range of different policy options in order to inform decisions. This can help to quantify and visualize the inherent trade-offs of pursuing one route rather than another in a world of finite resources.

Simulation models have been used to great effect for some time in the field of infectious diseases, modelling potential opportunities for interventions to reduce transmission in conditions such as HIV, or ebola in developing countries. But they have only recently begun to be utilized in high-income countries as an aid to addressing the increasing burden of lifestyle diseases. We now need to move the use of such modelling from the academic world to the big challenges and questions of our time, including LTCs and prevention.

Simulation modelling was recently used to review the health and economic effects of salt policy in the UK over the past decade. Prior to 2010, the UK was a world leader in salt policy, with the independent Food Standards Agency implementing a transparent approach to the reformulation of foods high in salt; the approach was closely monitored, with a threat of sanctions on industry if progress was not achieved. It worked. Salt consumption reduced by 15% over an eight-year period. This was estimated to have prevented 20,000 strokes, heart attacks, and heart failure cases a year and saved the UK economy more than £1.5 billion each year [9].

From 2011 the policy changed, becoming more relaxed; the threat of sanctions disappeared and the food industry marked their own homework. Previous progress stalled. Simulation modelling from Imperial College and the University of Liverpool found the switch in policy resulted in nearly 10,000 more cases of CVD. Looking forwards, the modelling showed this could also result in an additional 26,000 preventable CVD cases over the coming six years, costing the health service and wider economy an additional £1 billion [10].

This research demonstrates the potential of simulation modelling and the tremendous costs (both health and economic) involved in making the wrong choices. It shows that this type of scenario planning should be embedded into the machinery of any organization making decisions about the health of a population. Being able to compare interventions, and targeting those most at risk of ill health compared to a one-size-fits-all approach before decisions are made, can improve the services provided, saving both money and effort. It also helps in making the case for or against policies by modelling the different returns, health and economic, to all involved.

Modelling was front and centre across the world in the early phases of the response to COVID-19. The use of epidemiological modelling to map out what the pandemic might mean for case numbers, hospitalization, and deaths, as well as which interventions may be most effective in preventing virus transmission, informed government responses. Of course, all models have limitations and estimates carry great uncertainty warnings with them, for instance some of the UK models were initially based on approaches developed for influenza rather than coronaviruses. If this modelling was much broader than health, and demonstrated both the short- and long-term potential consequences of ill health on the economy (and the counterfactual, the potential benefits of total health), it would have enabled much more holistic and region-specific policy early and throughout the pandemic. This demonstrates, at the extreme, how in-silico modelling needs to be at the centre of government policy in the 21st century.

Using technology wisely

The advances that we should expect from predictive analytics over the coming years rely upon several factors: we must ask the questions that are most relevant to our pressing challenges; use comprehensive and representative data; and deliver answers through user-friendly tools and with wider support to enable the user to be empowered.

AI, along with many other emerging technologies, is a generalizable tool that provides the building blocks to address some of the biggest challenges in delivering health. Clinicians, patients, and the public must together help drive this agenda. In many ways, whether these technologies do transform healthcare for the better and if so, whether we all benefit, is down to each of us.

Central to making this happen is trust, and trust in technology amongst clinicians is increasing; a 2015 survey in the USA showed that 42% of doctors are willing to prescribe medications based on the results of consumer-operated diagnostic technologies [11]. Rather than a threat, clinicians must see AI as a tool that supports them to tackle the ever-increasing demand with decreasing resources.

As well as being accurate and easy to use, in order to integrate emerging technologies into clinical practice the algorithms must be understandable and interpretable to the users. Unlike many past processes that harnessed black-box approaches with opaque workings, going forward models need to have a high degree of transparency with the outputs interpretable to the full spectrum of users, because this has been shown to significantly increase engagement and adoption.

In addition, for algorithms to be useful, the data they learn from has to be representative of a population, to avoid the type of post-code lottery that happened with previous innovations in healthcare whereby inequalities in health actually worsened rather than improved. We all need to engage and understand the power of large datasets to improve healthcare hence health for others. Individuals can help by donating their data so that, anonymized, it can be used to develop technologies. But they need to trust the institutions and private sector companies that will be using that data, which in turn demands shared values and transparency on all sides.

To achieve the best outcomes, no matter how advanced the technologies become, we have to ask the most relevant questions. This requires those on the front line, the clinicians, to ask the right questions for technologies to provide answers to. Our citizens, too, have an important role to play in asking questions.

Technology has the power to put control of our (future) health in our own hands, through providing information and support to enable us to make healthier choices as well as redressing the balance in the management of LTCs between doctor and patient. In the wider context of our drivers of total health, technology can be an amplifier for us as individuals and as populations to shift the drivers of our health from being harmful to making healthy living easy.

References

1. Britnell M. *Human: solving the global workforce crisis in healthcare*. Oxford: Oxford University Press. March 2019.
2. Davies S. *Annual Report of the Chief Medical Officer, 2018: Health 2040—Better Health Within Reach*. Chapter 5. London: Department of Health and Social Care, 2018.
3. Hogan H, Zipfel R, Neuburger J, et al. Avoidability of hospital deaths and association with hospital-wide mortality ratios: retrospective case record review and regression analysis. *BMJ* 2015; 351:h3239
4. De Fauw J, Ledsam J, Romera-Paredes B, et al. Clinically applicable deep learning for diagnosis and referral in retinal disease. *Nat Med* **24**,1342–50 (2018). https://doi.org/10.1038/s41591-018-0107-6
5. Davies S. *Annual Report of the Chief Medical Officer, 2018: Health 2040—Better Health Within Reach*. Chapter 10. London: Department of Health and Social Care, 2018.
6. Hippisley-Cox J, Coupland C, Vinogradova Y, Robson J, May M, Brindle P. Derivation and validation of QRISK, a new cardiovascular disease risk score for the United Kingdom: prospective open cohort study. *BMJ*. 2007;335:136. doi:10.1136/bmj.39261.471806.55. pmid:17615182.
7. Gregg E, Cheng Y, Srinivasan M, et al. Trends in cause-specific mortality among adults with and without diagnosed diabetes in the USA: an epidemiological analysis of linked national survey and vital statistics data. *The* Lancet. 2018;391(10138):2430–40
8. Ahlqvist E, Storm P, Käräjämäki A, et al. Novel subgroups of adult-onset diabetes and their association with outcomes: a data-driven cluster analysis of six variables. *The Lancet Diabetes & Endocrinol.* 2018;6(5):361–69. doi:10.1016/S2213-8587(18)30051-2
9. MacGregor G, He F, Pombo-Rodrigues S. Food and the responsibility deal: how the salt reduction strategy was derailed. *BMJ* 2015;**350**.doi:10.1136/bmj.h1936
10. Laverty A, Kypridemos C, Seferidi P, et al. Quantifying the impact of the Public Health Responsibility Deal on salt intake, cardiovascular disease and gastric cancer burdens: interrupted time series and microsimulation study. *J Epidemiol Community Health*. 2019;73(9):881–87. doi:10.1136/jech-2018-211749
11. Williams B. Enabling better healthcare with artificial intelligence. PWC 2017.

9

So whose health is it? Time to value total health

Everything we value as humans depends on health. Our role within a family or social group is stronger if we are healthy; our prosperity relies on us being healthy enough to work; and, earlier in life, good health enables us to grow, develop, and realize our potential. The instinct to love and connect, the ability to find meaning, purpose, and dignity in work, equality and fairness in society, sustainability, literally everything is made possible, or at least easier, more enjoyable, and ultimately more satisfying if we are healthy.

So why is health seemingly not more precious to us? As a society, we do not seem to place a value on health that is concomitant with what it means to us in the 21st century, as individuals and as part of our wider community. We do not appreciate the currency of health, or how it underpins society and is central to our economy. Health should be recognized as an asset, something worth investing in, but at the moment, we see it—or rather illness, a lack of health—as a cost to individuals and society. Our so-called health system has become an expensive illness system, we resent the resources it requires, yet we run to it at the slightest provocation.

COVID-19 has taught us that health truly is our most untapped opportunity for collective prosperity, happiness, and fairness in the 21st century. Living well for longer removes the barriers holding back communities, improving opportunities for education, skills training, and work—good health can shift the life chances of individuals and communities. It is an investment, not a cost.

We have choices as we look to rebuild post-COVID-19. Our collective vulnerability to ill health has brought us together, and also shown us the stark realities of living in an unequal society. If we put good health at the centre of our collective recovery and rehabilitation from the pandemic, that would lay the foundations for a brighter future for us all.

When we ask people 'so whose health is it?' the almost invariable response is 'mine'. But how much control do we have of it? We believe the health of an individual is shaped by the genes they inherited from their parents, the

Whose Health Is It, Anyway? Dame Sally C. Davies and Jonathan Pearson-Stuttard, Oxford University Press (2021).
© Oxford University Press. DOI: 10.1093/oso/9780198863458.003.0009

family they are born into, the education they receive, and the opportunities they have. But all of this is shaped by the community, the society, and the environment in which they live. We have written in earlier chapters about the drivers of our health and particularly how the social drivers affect inequalities, but perhaps the least understood are the commercial drivers of our health. Many examples of these commercial drivers, including much of the food and drink industry, need to be incentivized to support good health or contribute through investment to improving health. We need policies where people everywhere recognize we are all in this together, that health is an asset to all of us and health is put above profit. This means we need a 'whole society approach' [1] which includes the private sector recognizing the need for them to innovate in order to incentivize total health, whilst protecting their profits. Everyone in society will benefit from working together to make this happen.

In this final chapter, we review some of the key issues and describe a multi-pronged approach that starts from a true understanding of the value of health to individuals and to society. We outline the entities and processes that could underpin a new total health ecosystem, one that values health and that could serve to take us into a happier and more prosperous future (see Fig. 9.1).

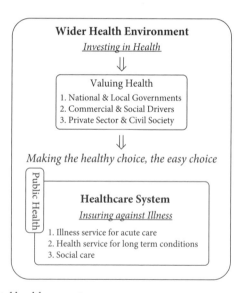

Fig. 9.1 The total health ecosystem

The need for change is clearer than ever

COVID-19 has brought deep-rooted and entrenched inequalities in drivers of our health and health outcomes to the fore; the pandemic has affected all of us, but not equally, and in ways that are predictable. The most deprived—financially and socially—are consistently more vulnerable to early death and disability. We have known for decades of the inequalities in health outcomes and that the most deprived 10% of men and women live nearly 10 years less than the most affluent 10%.

We know too that this is avoidable—that if cancer survival rates were equal across all sectors of society, 10,000 lives would be saved over just five years [2]—but COVID-19 laid bare the inequalities in an unrelenting and brutal manner. The most deprived 20% were more than twice as likely to die from COVID-19 than the most affluent, and some Black, Asian, and Minority Ethnic (BAME) groups were found to have as much as three times the risk of the general population, with much of this increased risk down to things that could be changed if we as a society chose to make a fairer system, one that valued total health and made the healthy choice the easy choice for all.

Looking ahead, we can see that, unless we take action now, the differential effects of the pandemic on the drivers of health are likely to become even greater. Education (school, higher education, and adult skill training) and work combine with health to shape the future prospects of individuals and communities. We knew before COVID-19 that poor education and poor work opportunities cluster in communities with poor health, and that health has become a bigger predictor of work opportunities than ever before. The gap has been made much bigger in just a few months. The closure of schools has amplified educational inequalities, with those in deprived areas falling behind those in more affluent areas because they have had less access to online options due to a combination of lack of teaching resources and the availability and affordability of the necessary technology.

Inequality in employment opportunities are also increasing. The lowest earning 10% were seven times more likely to work in sectors that closed during lockdown in Spring 2020, and many of these sectors will be slower to re-open, if they do at all, and apparently with greater redundancies. Tolerating the lockdown itself was much more difficult in more deprived communities—denser housing, less outdoor space, having to use public transport, a greater sense of uncertainty, and lack of agency all contributed to worsening conditions for the most deprived, in turn making them more vulnerable to the disease and its wider effects.

Modern societies often behave in ways that do not value health and even harm health. At the most extreme, we have created markets that incentivize selling products that actively harm our health, such as tobacco, which again shines a harsh light on inequality. Smoking rates are higher in deprived communities, and, apart from the fact that smokers are at greater risk of contracting a number of diseases and cancers as a result of their habit, we now know that they are not only more likely to become infected with COVID-19, but are also more likely to suffer severe symptoms. Many countries, including the UK, have shown how we can work separately and together to reduce tobacco consumption, but without valuing health over illness in general, efforts will remain patchy and uneven.

Our vulnerability to ill health through an environment promoting unhealthy behaviour and failing to value the role of health across societies and nations left us collectively frail when COVID-19 hit, particularly with obesity, diabetes and related illnesses. But we do not have to continue to entrench inequalities across society generation after generation. We do not have to remain vulnerable to shocks like COVID-19, it is possible to change. As we invest to rebuild society, we have to look carefully at how we value health across our entire environment, not just at the point of delivery of acute services. We have to understand better the multiple drivers of our health and how the changing world around us affects our health, and we have to find a better way to measure health rather than quantifying illness. Above all, we have to find ways to incentivize rebuilding health across all sectors, from the private sector to civil society, and to incentivize health as an investment in our collective resilience and future prosperity.

The wider health environment

We have seen that there are multiple drivers of health, beyond simply what is provided by healthcare services. Although frequently interlinked, we have discussed them in the contexts of commercial and social drivers, and also explored the ways that shared values based on mutual benefit can provide a way forward.

The environment around us makes it all too easy to be unhealthy. Health has always played second fiddle when profits are concerned, so it is not surprising that 'profits before people' is a familiar expression. If we truly appreciated the prosperity that health brings, our society would not allow the cheapest most accessible food to be the most obesogenic. Nor would we see the soft drinks industry levy, an innovative policy that is held up time and time again as an exemplar of how to foster healthier products without harming profits, as a one-off. This would be the norm. The soft drinks industry levy in the UK demonstrated that healthier products do not necessarily have to be less profitable products, and innovative companies can make profits without damaging health, or at least reducing this impact. This approach could be applied to salt in processed or prepared foods, or the government could institute a public health tax on prepacked goods, as in Hungary on levels of calorie, sugar, and salt [1], or indeed on non-essential food and drinks.

The prosperity of businesses is also reliant on the health of their workforce and local communities. It is rare for companies to truly invest in the health of their workers and families, even though there are a few great examples from our own past and around the world. But for every company that demonstrates the true meaning of corporate social responsibility, there are many more that do not.

Civil society creates the external environment in which we live, and we must all take more action, realizing that we do have the power to make changes. We have seen that some of the biggest drivers of our health and inequalities, such as housing and income, are not in fact fixed, unchangeable 'determinants', but can be as modifiable as the food we eat each day—if we choose to value total health and make changes. One stark example was the housing of all homeless individuals during the first wave of COVID-19; taking them off the streets across England could change the lives of many long-term.

Making this happen means government policies are required that put health and living well for longer, adding life to years not just years to life. A recent report from the McKinsey Global Institute attempted to quantify this health dividend. They estimated that through applying interventions that we know work, the global disease burden could be reduced by 40% and that this in turn could add $12 trillion, or 8%, to global GDP by 2040 [3]. They found the social benefits could be much bigger, as much as $100 trillion globally, and help reduce income inequality. Clearly this will pay off and investment is essential, but it is about more than just investment. It is about a shift in philosophy so we all value health, and so that the different parts of government are joined up and working together to deliver the opportunity of health for everyone fairly and sustainably.

A new way to measure—and value—total health: the National Health Index

We do not measure health, we count illness. Instead of indicators of wellness and well-being, we measure incidences of illnesses, numbers of treatments and, on occasions, outcomes. Governments often rely on life expectancy to see how they are doing—but this measure does little to capture peoples' health in the years lived, it fails to recognize the intrinsic links between health and wealth, and life expectancy is historical, so the numbers are always far behind the curve. This means that the big issues are left as tomorrow's problem for someone else to deal with. To review and assess our services we rely on audit and physical inspections across the health and care system, which are also backward-looking. This ignores the wealth of data and digital approaches that could help anticipate and avoid difficulties, instead, retrospective sanctions are handed out.

We need a new approach to health that goes beyond the NHS, and which puts front and centre the pivotal role of total health in our prosperity as a nation going forwards. An approach that helps us to look ahead, build on best practice, and plan for a better future. We must recognize and reposition health within society as the opportunity that it is.

In the Annual Report of the Chief Medical Officer, 2018, authored by us, we introduced the concept of a Composite Health Index. This idea is rooted in repositioning total health as an asset to a nation, rather than ill health being a drain. The index, currently being developed by the Office for National Statistics (ONS) with a beta version expected in Autumn 2020, captures the complex factors that represent total health in order to track progress to a healthier future.

Historically, by focusing on the traditional outcome measures such as life expectancy mentioned above, we have been unable to identify the key drivers of our stock of health as a nation, nor to flag and intervene before it is too late. The Composite Health Index instead recognizes total health to be an opportunity for economic prosperity and happiness, both nationally and locally. It provides a set of metrics that should sit next to the gross domestic product, GDP, and now is the time to rename it the National Health Index (NHI).

The NHI has three layers: healthy people, healthy lives, and healthy places. The first includes data such as infant mortality and cancer survival; healthy lives includes the prevalence of overweight, obesity, and smoking, along with factors like the availability of stable employment that pays a living wage; and healthy places incorporates the wider environment, including local air pollution, access to green spaces, cycling infrastructure, and housing quality. Importantly, health inequalities are captured at each level.

Alongside tracking the stock of health, the NHI must have a policy impact tool using simulation modelling to visualize the potential health, economic, and equity impacts of policies from across government (national and local) to truly put health at the centre of decision making.

By collectively valuing health, we can then transform the wider health environment to one that invests in health. We recommend that this is underpinned by three innovative new societal contracts: new shared values between the private sector, civil society and our nation's total health; a new 21st century public health system that includes monitoring with surveillance and health security; and an expanded NHS that provides a health and care system that encompasses acute and chronic illness along with social care, truly there for us from the cradle to the grave.

Shared prosperity if we value total health

COVID-19 has shown us that the future prospects of all of society, including businesses and the health of communities and nations, are inextricably linked. We need a whole society approach. The public and private sectors, individuals, and governments must recognize that health is a shared value. It is our most untapped opportunity for prosperity, and is also an asset for individuals, for employers, and for society.

We must partner better together, building on this shared value. The public and private sectors should look after the health of their employees, both physical and mental, and also pay a contribution towards the public's health where they cannot make provision. They should also contribute to total health by reaching out to workers' families and the local communities in which they operate, creating a wider health environment that fosters total health—an investment that will pay off for all.

This is not such a radical move, instead it is a natural next step from recent trends. The Public Services (Social Value) Act came into force in the UK in 2013 and required commissioners across the public sector to consider social and environmental well-being as well as economic factors when procuring contracts. This act fundamentally aims to get the most value from public spending, acknowledging that value is much a wider concept than solely short-term cost. The next phase includes employing local residents or targeting younger unemployed people, requiring contractors to pay living wages, and procuring with local voluntary and social enterprise groups. This is now more pressing than ever as we rebuild post COVID-19, and the private sector must play its part.

The NHS at the local level cannot be exempt from contributing to the health of their workforce and families either. The NHS is the biggest employer in the UK and should be leading the way in valuing health. From promoting active travel to ensuring only healthy food and drink are available on site, and supporting weight reduction, vaccination programmes, and alcohol, drug and smoking cessation services, the NHS could do so much to look after the health of their own workforce, and reach out through them to their families and communities.

Investing in the new public health for the 21st century

The COVID-19 pandemic has reminded us all how crucial public health is to preventing ill health, but for decades total health as we have called it has been undervalued and not given enough resources in communities and across the nation.

The Public Health system has a larger role than that of promoting and improving the health of individuals and inclusivity. It also needs to underpin how we collectively value health in the wider health environment, and to work with the NHS around health security, which includes infectious diseases, whether tackling prevention or dealing with outbreaks, epidemics, and pandemics. We should continue to fund our health security needs from taxation, as an insurance for the population—albeit at higher levels of funding than now. Not only will Public Health have to work closely with our 21st century healthcare system, but a lot of this work will be done locally, particularly around improving total health, and therefore it needs to be delivered by local communities and local government.

The new 21st century Public Health alongside the NHS must both embrace data to inform decision making and weave this into all aspects of health across communities. The National Health Index will reveal the health needs of communities, as well as that of the whole nation, to shed light on where to invest for a more prosperous tomorrow. This must start with a nationwide approach to tackling some of the big issues, for instance using robust data to push through a radical re-pricing of the commercial drivers holding back our health—food and beverages, alcohol, and tobacco—to reflect the true cost to society and incentivize industry to innovate and make their products healthier.

Most of the private sector contributes positively to society but, like all of us, must shift to valuing health more in the 21st century to realize the dividends this can bring. Many businesses could do more, from providing mental health support to health improvement. There is a small minority, though, that actively harm health—those behind the leading commercial drivers of ill health, such as tobacco, alcohol, and unhealthy food.

All companies should 'play or pay' to invest in communities and the total health of the nation. They should make a financial contribution to the new public health dependent on their health impacts, profits, and footprint in the country. We can no longer accept private companies, particularly multinationals, freeloading and not recognizing their responsibilities to either their workers or to the societies where they sell their goods and services. Where the profits arise from products and services that contribute to ill health, they should pay nationally towards improving public health – into the National Public Health Investment Fund. The payments could then be offset against a company's contribution to the health of their workers and communities at the local, regional, and national level. If, for instance, food companies voluntarily reduced portion-size on unhealthy food and drink, reduced the number of calories each portion contained, and adopted more ethical marketing, then they could offset this against their contribution to the new public health. These two elements combined, play or pay, will enable us to build healthy communities and have real and significant funding to invest in the health of those communities.

The pandemic has given us a glimmer of the integral role of Public Health, as well as the consequences of not valuing prevention. The 2012 Health and Social Care Act in England putting public health into local authority held great promise for influencing the health of communities, licensing, and true population health, yet local authorities have not been supported to act on it. The mismatch between funding and where benefits accrue, alongside ever tightening budgets, has prevented progress, often in the areas of highest health need, worsening the postcode lottery and hardening social inequalities for another generation. Meanwhile, the clinical services transferred, including contraception and sexual health, drugs, alcohol, and smoking cessation services, have deteriorated in many places. In the future, ensuring our health security both locally and nationally through the new National Institute for Health Protection must not be compromised. Too often we start with the system entrenching complexity and erecting artificial boundaries and barriers based on whether the care is, in the community, hospital, nursing home or the individual's own home—but what matters is our health. We must start with the patient or the citizen, recognize that health is no longer personal and how it has changed, and then design a system that keeps all of us living well for longer, and rewards all of those involved in making it happen with real time data at its heart.

The fourth industrial revolution of data and digital technology has dramatically altered the way we live, from banking and booking holidays 24/7 to Face Timing family and friends wherever they are in the world. Yet we have been slow to embrace these technologies in our healthcare system. Again, COVID-19 has shown us how this can be done, and what might have taken years has been adopted in days, from easy electronic repeat prescriptions to video medical consultations and complex logistics data to assist ordering and delivery of life-saving supplies to hospitals. We need to protect, build, and invest in these advances and welcome the disruption that can lead to better services. We must make the NHS a hotbed for digital innovation that works for everyone and bring individuals with us, contributing to and benefiting from data-driven services in real time. We should be using data rather than inspection to review, support, and improve our health services.

Alongside shaping the wider health environment that underpins our collective good of valuing health, Public Health services must also leverage the potential of technology to embed early diagnostics across communities, and screening programmes that are smart and proportionate to risk, including using modern technologies such as genomics with personalized risk scores. We need to extend the reach of these programmes across communities, helping all to benefit. Modern science and technology must be the foundation of all our services. Getting this right will help us to improve the health of the poorest fastest, making levelling up a reality for millions.

Insuring and ensuring a 21st century healthcare system treating illness and driving total health

Our NHS was set up, funded by taxation, as an impressively progressive integral part of the welfare state, but it has become an illness system and COVID-19 has demonstrated that it has poor resilience. Our NHS has been there supporting us in our moment of need, however, the illness model it was founded on has not helped us to live well in the community, and this includes its many employees. The NHS has been muddling through, getting patched up when there are problems but largely continuing as the illness service it has become. We can look at it as insuring against illness and funding treatment through taxation, but we have not invested in the dual purpose of both treating illness and fostering total health. Nor have we truly invested in the infrastructure, training, and culture we need to harness modern digital services to support the public, patients, clinicians, and managers as most other sectors have done. Sadly, we also know that too often people are harmed through their interactions with our hospitals and community services, as a result of catching infections, the side effects of treatment, and even mistakes.

If we reposition health as an asset we can have a new proactive and more resilient NHS and a wider system for Public Health. We must recognize one purpose of the NHS is to treat ill health and recognize that a lot of activity within it is transactional, but we must not lose sight of the central primary purpose being also about humanity, relationships, and fairness. We have to invest for a new accessible, respectful, and dignified service with people at the centre—a resilient illness and expanded healthcare system. Coalescing around the individual needs of each and every citizen, the healthcare system must increase the stock of health in communities through each interaction.

Our 21st century NHS must be a healthcare system that embraces three parallel interconnected functions and services. The first builds on the illness system that deals with our acute illnesses, the second is a true health system that helps us to live in good health and with chronic conditions, and the third is a social care system that provides dignity and comfort from the cradle to the grave, as the NHS was initially founded to do. These three parallel systems require different structures, incentives, and even workforces, but must work synergistically together and focus on and around the person.

The illness system builds on the best of what the NHS was founded to do and has done for more than 70 years. From symptoms to rehabilitation, it covers acute illness, non-infectious conditions such as strokes, and road traffic accidents as well as acute infectious diseases, such as COVID-19. It has to be a truly national system that integrates research and learning to deliver high-quality, safe care for everyone wherever they are, and gets them back into their communities without delay. The workforce needs to be specialist and skilled, backed up by effective technologies that optimize their time as well as treatment for the patient. At the foundation must be data moving seamlessly with the patient.

Our NHS has risen to the COVID-19 challenge really well but we now know that both hospitals and care homes have been centres of infection. In addition, many patients in the community have been deterred from using the NHS because of the risk of catching infections and the strong message to 'stay at home'. The delays in treatment of chronic conditions such as cancer look to be putting back years of progress on cancer survival rates. It is clear for all to see that we must have an illness system that is resilient enough for subsequent waves of COVID-19 and future pandemics and that this is likely to require separation of routine care from acute and responsive care. The basis of separation for protection, as with all infection control measures, needs to be effective, and to provide continuity of care from first symptom to rehabilitation and convalescence.

We now know that COVID-19 is transmitted through close proximity, touching, droplets, and aerosols, as well as through faces and families. Although many infected persons are mildly affected or even have no symptoms, particularly the young, others require hospitalization, and respiratory and other organ support, which has a high death rate, particularly in the elderly or those with long-term conditions. We are also increasingly seeing the long-term toll, including neurological, cardiac, renal, and musculo-skeletal problems in some who have been infected with COVID-19 that will require specialist intensive rehabilitation and support for months and maybe years to come.

We believe that the NHS should run all clinical services, because we have seen that services transferred via public health grants to local authorities have not been applied consistently and have been subject to cuts. Despite worthy intentions, this has had unintended consequences and has, for instance, resulted in a postcode lottery for contraception services for women, and smoking cessation and substance misuse programmes. Public Health has often not been able to deliver clinical services because the local authorities, themselves trying to do more with fewer resources, do not accrue the benefit of outcomes, such as reduced pressure on NHS services or complications during treatment, directly—an important commodity in a world of priorities and choices.

As well as its core illness service, our 21st century healthcare system needs to develop an effective health empowering service for patients with long-term conditions to help them remain as well and independent as possible for as long as possible. Patients need non-intrusive home monitoring, applications to help, nudges to remind, and the data all brought together for and in their health records—easily accessible and actionable information for patients and clinicians. The service for long-term conditions needs to be close to the patient and only use hospitals when that is the best option for the patient, or when specialist interventions are needed. Those who are not ill need not be in or visiting hospitals; healthcare systems for long-term conditions should be local systems, acknowledging how health needs vary across communities, and that physical, mental, and social health needs are equal. The workforce here must be more generalist than in the illness service, to reflect the multimorbid nature of populations and as multimorbidity continues to increase, building on the strength of our GPs.

The NHS has made great strides in minimizing the relative gap in life expectancy for society as a whole over the past 70 years, but to reduce the gap in healthy life, and the opportunity this will bring throughout life, the principles of the NHS must be extended to social care. Hence the third stream of this new model is a National Care Service that brings dignity and fairness to ageing and all of those requiring social care across the nation, based on the principles of the NHS.

At its inception, the NHS was intended to provide care and dignity in illness from cradle to grave. It has often struggled with our final portion of life, but now it is from cradle to care home, amplifying all the inequalities felt throughout life, which in turn worsens the final few years of life and increases the costs of care. The National Care Service must be born, not separate to, but as part of the NHS—no more barriers, no more excuses—and continuing care must be simple and seamless for patients and families, putting them, their dignity, and total health at the centre. Again, we have to ensure that we insure for our care in later years, whether through direct taxation or other insurance for those who can pay.

Health and social care should be managed and coordinated locally, with the incentives uniting the dozens of stakeholders around the long-term health and wellness of each individual. The hospital should only be visited when ill—health belongs in the community and as part of our daily lives. From having vaccinations before or after doing your weekly shop in the supermarket to blood pressure checks in the pharmacy or at home, maintaining good health should be the default, easy option.

Alongside creating these clear, parallel yet interlinked services to treat, deliver health, and underpin social care, the NHS must shift its culture too, and embrace technology, science, and innovation. Health is a collaborative endeavour, with academia, life sciences, and the technology industry all contributing, but our British system is not alone in making it easier to work in silos than to collaborate and innovate collectively. Without sorting out these tribal and philosophical problems between the private sector, the NHS, academia, community partners, and local authorities, we will not embrace science in the way we must if we are, for instance, to bring genomics into our national screening programmes effectively and early to save later suffering. Collaboration is also needed within the healthcare system itself. All of our services need to be data-driven, with the data moving with the patients and service users but also, as we have seen during the pandemic, aggregated and used for learning and research to improve outcomes system-wide and underpinning effective logistics and management. Data hoarding has to become history.

A National Bank for Health

We have to think through how we can structure these three services. We need also to ensure accountability and full oversight of the whole health system to realize the opportunity that health brings. The whole system consists of two areas: the wider health environment, where the opportunity of health must be incentivized and invested in; and the health and care system, the parallel, interlinked services that act as an insurance, an extension of the underpinning values of the NHS.

We also have to think how these functions and services can be funded and at a considerably higher level than presently. We have already made the distinction between insuring for health funded from general taxation and investing for the public's health—our most untapped opportunity. Post COVID-19 there is clearly acceptance among the public that we need to spend more on the NHS, that is increasing our insurance to deliver better care for those who are ill, better screening, vaccination, and clinical services, as well as protecting our staff effectively.

Health and investing in total health should be looked at like long-term asset management across a 25-year horizon based firmly on the return on investment (ROI). The assets should be invested for ROI, in other words to ensure total health and in turn prosperity for the nation, delivering a recurring dividend to everyone in the country. According to the Mckinsey Global Institute, every $1 spent on health would result in between $2-$4 economic return [3]. The judgements, or measures, against which assets are invested must reflect the value of health—living well for longer rather than simpler measures such as life expectancy, relating to many facets of health in the round, and including modifiable risk factors and social determinants of health as well as health outcomes—that is by using the NHI.

Economic growth is central to a nation's prosperity, and this is driven in most countries by a Central Bank that performs a range of activities, from overseeing monetary policy to setting the framework and targets for measures such as inflation and employment. The primary function of the Bank of England, for instance, is to maintain monetary stability, oversee the financial stability of the UK financial system, and help to build a strong and stable economy for the public it serves.

Can we transfer that concept to health? We now realize that health is as crucial an asset as currency for our future prosperity. Hence we propose a National Bank for Health, independent of government, that can function as an oversight body and do for health what the Bank of England does for monetary policy (see Table 9.1) including managing the National Public Health Investment Fund.

The National Bank for Health would help us to realize the opportunity of health in the 21st century by providing the governance and framework we need to ensure that we collectively value health across society, recognizing that this will pay off. The primary function would be to build our stock of health systematically and comprehensively across both the nation and the healthcare system to ensure at all times and in all places it is made easier to be healthy and deliver prosperity. It would capture our stock of health measured by the National Health Index and take account of the time-lag for the dividends of many drivers of health to come to fruition. It would create a framework for health, recommend insurance, investment levels, and allocations for health based on data, manage the National Public Health Investment Fund, and review the functioning of the overall system, especially at the interfaces between the parts. Importantly, the National Bank for Health would regulate and supervise investments to deliver better health.

The National Bank for Health would hold each stakeholder to account and oversee the stability of the UK system both for the wider health environment and the healthcare system—putting the health of people and communities first. Across the wider health environment, the National Bank for Health would set the framework for us all to play our part in valuing health, and for the Government plus private sector—local or national—to do this on our behalf.

With a National Bank for Health, a metric capturing our stock of health (NHI) and the new National Public Health Fund for Investment, we will then truly be in a position to value health. The NHI can be used as the backbone to estimate the impacts—positive or negative that each actor is having on our wider health environment, underpinning the play or pay mechanism. It would show

Table 9.1 Functions of the National Bank for Health compared to the Bank of England

Bank of England	National Bank of Health
Independent of Government	Independent of Government
Look after the gold reserve	Look after health as a national asset including inequalities in health
Maintain monetary stability and oversee financial stability of UK financial system	Maintain improvement in the population's health, measured by the National Health Index Oversee the stability of the expanded healthcare system.
Manage monetary policy and maintain money supply	Manage stable spending on healthcare Set the framework for contributions for the 'play or pay' system to value health across the wider health environment
Ensure smooth electronic payments	Ensure smooth data flows, transfers, surveillance, and inter-operability across the healthcare system
Reduce system financial risk and ensure banks are safe and sound	Ensure institutions across the healthcare system are safe and sound
Financial policy committee	**Health Policy Committee**
Macroprudential regulation	Review return on investment over longer time horizon and resilience regulation across the healthcare system
Set interest rates	Set the contributions for private sector 'play or pay' system to value total health across the wider health environment and framework for the National Public Health Investment Fund Set the national/local split of funding and powers for the population's health Set the framework for outcomes-based commissioning across local health economies according to health (Local Health Indices)
Prudential Regulation Authority	**Health Regulation Authority**
Microprudential regulation	Ensure all parts of the healthcare system act safely and work collaboratively in the interests of their local population's total health using a data-driven approach
Supervision and stress testing of financial institutions	Supervision and stress-testing of healthcare system institutions (including local authorities), programmes, health security, and actors

the role of government more transparently, bringing to light how decisions made in non-health departments today will influence our stock of health in years to come, and what that means for communities across the country.

The National Health Index needs and will have local indices too, providing a framework for local reimbursements across the NHS and wider health economy—investing directly in health, and continuing to insure for the more comprehensive illnesses across our lifetimes. Interactive and dynamic local Health Indices will give more tools and more weight to health locally, making it easier to build healthier environments and bring to light the measures with the biggest returns to populations and on what timescale. All in the knowledge that the shared value of health will bring prosperity.

The National Bank for Health would also oversee the structure and implementation of an interoperable digital framework across the whole health ecosystem—much broader than just the NHS—that encourages innovators, public and private, to develop their products in the UK and deliver the best care to our patients, whilst also ensuring that a patient's record follows them, whether they are in primary care in Dorset, or social care in Newcastle-upon-Tyne. But this must also go much further: disease surveillance, screening, and testing must all be based on the latest science, digitized, and real-time to better inform national and local preventative policies.

Banks, building societies, and insurers are regulated by the Prudential Regulation Authority (PRA), a part of the Bank of England that uses data to ensure firms act safely and reduces the chances of them getting into financial difficulty. Our regulation and inspections of hospitals and the NHS remain stuck in the past—clipboard inspections that disrupt day-to-day work, often hitting morale and camaraderie in an already stretched workforce. The regulatory framework has not done enough to improve the quality of care, nor reduce inequalities across the NHS. The National Bank for Health should, like the PRA, co-ordinate the use of data to identify what is comparable across hospitals and what is not, encouraging the sharing of learning, innovation, and success, and supporting and identifying where and how healthcare can be improved. Better healthcare is better for the patient and the bottom line.

Incentivizing total health and the National Public Health Investment Fund

Our total health is not just an absence of physical illness, but also includes our mental and social well-being. There are multiple ways in which we can incentivize total health, from how we fund acute illness services to the ways we encourage and nudge all of society, including the private sector, to acknowledge their share in total health and contribute accordingly.

We spend 9.6% of our GDP on health, that is insuring us all for illness. This is middle of the pack in the OECD countries, but second lowest amongst the G7 group. Polling shows that we are willing to pay more in tax towards the NHS. We could also look at the wealth inequalities that now exist between some segments of the retiring baby boomer generation and the generations coming behind them, and review the national insurance contributions for those who are older than the state pension age but continue to work into their 70s to help fun our National Care Service.

The key new funding to improve and deliver total health must come as investment from both taxation and the private sector—health is our collective opportunity for a brighter future. COVID-19 has forced the private sector to recognize the adverse impact of poor health both on their workforce and on their bottom line, and now is the time for them to contribute to improving public health locally and nationally. As well as direct levies or 'public health taxes' on products adding to the National Public Health Investment Fund, the private sector can also contribute through how companies look after their employees, their families, and their communities—the 'play' element of investment. This is not about stifling innovation, nor putting barriers up for businesses, especially small and medium size enterprises. Those with the broadest shoulders, or those actively harming our health, must contribute the most, manifesting the new shared values and shared responsibilities every day, not just when we have an emergency. All in the knowledge that valuing health will pay off.

The National Bank for Health can set the framework for this approach, and the contribution of a company to the total health of their employees, their community, and/or the nation, can be assessed against the framework. If it reaches the agreed level, the company has 'played' and that is their part in valuing health. Companies that do not meet the agreed level would pay into the National Public Health Investment Fund, which in turn will invest in supporting the nation's public health. This fund for total health could be spent nationally, including on social marketing to promote health or, for example 'essential food vouchers' [1] for those with greatest need, particularly children. The National Public Health Investment Fund could also in part be devolved to be allocated locally according to priorities and challenges that often vary considerably across the country. Inherent in this model would be the need to assess the contribution or negative impact of companies' products and their supply chains to the health of the public, and analysis of factors such as whether the company provides physical and mental health benefits and a secure and stable income for its employees.

We also need a step change in the pricing of the environment which dominates our health behaviours. The soft drinks industry levy has shown what is possible—a radical redrawing of pricing of foods and drinks that incentivized innovation across the industry. Those that do not innovate and create healthier products should face increased levies so that they pay a fairer contribution to the ill health, and poorer work and learning opportunities that their products create. The National Bank for Health would allocate the investment funds of the National Public Health Investment Fund nationally or locally depending on both need and potential ROI to deliver total health. Locally, the money could be used by local government and communities to support priority needs, which could include expanding successful programmes like the healthy start programme for lower income families.

We know that we need innovative financing mechanisms for health to increase levels of investment. The private sector having to play or pay is one idea. Another option is to borrow the concept of sustainable debt instruments from the environmental sector. These are loans made to institutions with the interest rate tied to a specific green/sustainable key performance indicator (KPI). The loan is tied to a particular use (e.g. developing wind farms, developing social housing) and if the KPI is achieved in any given year, then the institution receives a lower rate of interest for that year, i.e. a financial discount. If the KPI is not met, the institution pays a higher rate, directly incentivizing innovation to achieve the agreed KPI. In a similar fashion, loans for total health or health impact bonds could be for activities like developing active transport measures or preventing falls in the homes of our elders, with the interest rates set by the National Bank for Health related to beneficial measured outcomes.

Citizen pressure has also led to the increasing adoption of socially responsible investing, and this offers another prime opportunity for health economies. The National Bank for Health could tie the rate of interest on loans and bonds to the contribution to health that a business, public body, or government makes. Getting this right would reduce the cost of the healthcare system, freeing up public sector money for other areas.

Whose health is it, anyway?

In this book we have set out to explain why health is central to our collective prosperity and underpins everyone's happiness in the 21st century. So the answer to the question, 'Whose health is it, anyway?' is, 'everyone's': ours as individuals, collectively as communities, and society all at the same time.

Health is vital for each of us and for all of us, and throughout this book we have described how our health and the factors that influence our health are less under our control as individuals and citizens than most people recognize. The fact that so much that influences our most valuable commodity, and in turn our ability to learn, work, and love, is in the hands of others—who are rarely incentivized and generally do not share our vision of valuing health—is a frightening prospect.

We believe that COVID-19 has demonstrated that altruism, human kindness, and caring about the delivery of healthcare and fairness in our society exists, just as bestselling author Rutger Bregman has recently set out in his book, *Humankind* [4]. Now we need to use our new understanding and collective power to democratize the opportunity of health and rebuild after COVID-19 with the biggest leap forward for our society since the NHS was set up in 1948, shifting our healthcare systems from importers of illness to exporters of health. Everyone should be working to make the healthy choice the easy choice for all of us. All of this underpinned by the knowledge that valuing health will pay off.

We can see an opportunity to take some of the politics out of our health ecosystem even whilst recognizing that politicians will always be accountable for such a large and growing portion of GDP. For this reason, we propose the creation of a partner to the independent Bank of England, the independent National Bank for Health. The National Health Index will be to the National Bank for Health what GDP is to the Bank of England. In addition, it would adopt data-driven regulation of the health system and set the framework for and distribute the National Public Health Investment Fund to increase our stock of health. Valuing health today will pay off for us all in the future.

We all have a voice but, those with large footprints and big platforms have an opportunity to play their part in building a better future for all. We have outlined how, through the digital age and social movements incorporating new power, the tide is turning and that, collectively, citizens united around a clear purpose have the potential to drive change faster and further than ever before. We saw an example of this in June 2020, when Marcus Rashford, a footballer for Manchester United and England, engineered a government U-turn that the Opposition could not achieve, and many thought impossible. Using his platform, backed by millions of supporters on social media, Rashford sent an open letter to government asking them to extend free school meals throughout the summer holidays for the most deprived children, to avoid worsening food poverty. Within 48 hours, the £120m COVID Summer Food Fund for 1.3 million school children was announced. Feeding those children will be feeding our future, not just theirs.

Health is for and belongs to all of us, it is our platform to a brighter, more prosperous, happy, and fair future. But we all know now is the time for actions, not just words. With every day that goes by, the opportunity of health and the prosperity, happiness, and fairness it promises passes by, too. We hope through this book and by sharing our ideas that we can start a national conversation on the sort of health ecosystem we need in the future, how it can be funded and run, and importantly how it will be held accountable. We hope everyone can and will join in the debate.

References

1. Hochlaf D, Thomas C. *The whole society approach: Making a giant leap on childhood health*. London: IPPR. August 2020. https://www.ippr.org/research/publications/the-whole-society-approach
2. Exarchakou A, et al. In: Davies SC. *Annual Report of the Chief Medical Officer, 2018, Health 2040 Better Health Within Reach*. London: Department of Health and Social Care, 2018.
3. Remes J, Linzer K, Singhal S, et al. *Prioritizing Health: A prescription for prosperity*. *McKinsey Global Institute*. 08 July 2020: https://www.mckinsey.com/industries/healthcare-systems-and-services/our-insights/prioritizing-health-a-prescription-for-prosperity
4. Bregman R. *Humankind: A Hopeful History*. London: Bloomsbury. 2020.

Index